W0246443

"Dr. Jessica Stone provides a great resource for understanding the complexities of new technologies in mental health. Useful to both digital natives as well as therapists less experienced with tech, the book offers a multidisciplinary framework for empowering professionals to embrace today's digital solutions and customize them for patients' needs".

Valentino Megale, *PhD, CEO Softcare Studios*

"*Technology in Mental Health* takes the mental health professional on a journey—a mindful and educated journey. This resource gives the therapist a clear understanding of the 'why' of technology in mental health with a thorough review of grounded mental health processes and their application within technology-based practices. The book further highlights the 'how,' educating professionals in how to implement the intersection of technology and mental health. If you have been curious or are needing validation for the use of technology in mental health care, this is your new resource."

Robert Jason Grant, *EdD, RPT-S, author and creator of AutPlay® Therapy*

"Innovation often dances with fear of the unknown. Dr. Stone carves a clear path in this essential foundational text about our inevitable transformation into the field of digital mental health. She normalizes and defines our space of human discomfort, dives into the crux of our mind and biology to eloquently explore our inner workings, educates us on essential digital ethical and cultural considerations, and guides us to deep understanding of how digital technologies can truly align with us be utilized as part of mental healthcare practice. Dr. Stone and her work are a true gift to our profession and the future of mental healthcare."

Rachel A. Altvater, *PsyD, RPT-S*

Technology in Mental Health

Technology in Mental Health focuses on the responsible integration of technology into therapy in a world affected by COVID. Author Jessica Stone discusses the effects of the pandemic on the field of mental health with historical fundamentals and possible future implications. Chapters also explore legal and ethical considerations, as well as educational and supervision needs. Seasoned and new clinicians alike will find valuable information in these pages as they progress from traditional to modern to post-COVID mental health treatment.

Jessica Stone, PhD, RPT-S, is a licensed psychologist in Colorado. She has been a practitioner, professor, presenter, mentor, and author for more than 30 years. Dr. Stone's interest in therapeutic digital tools has culminated in clinical mental health use and research for mental health, medical, and crisis settings.

Routledge Focus on Mental Health

Routledge Focus on Mental Health presents short books on current topics, linking in with cutting-edge research and practice.

Titles in the series:

Psychoanalysis and Euripides' Suppliant Women: A Tragic Reading of Politics
Sotiris Manolopoulos

The Gifts We Receive from Animals: Stories to Warm the Heart
Lori R. Kogan

James Joyce and the Internal World of the Replacement Child
Mary Adams

Analytic Listening in Clinical Dialogue: Basic Assumptions
Dieter Bürgin, Angelika Staehle, Kerstin Westhoff, and Anna Wyler von Ballmoos

Treatment for Body-Focused Repetitive Behaviors: An Integrative Psychodynamic Approach
Stacy K. Nakell

Psychoanalysis and the Act of Artistic Creation: A Look at the Unconscious Dynamics of Creativity
Luís Manuel Romano Delgado

Technology in Mental Health: Foundations for Clinical Use
Jessica Stone

For a full list of titles in this series, please visit https://www.routledge.com/Routledge-Focus-on-Mental-Health/book-series/RFMH

Technology in Mental Health
Foundations of Clinical Use

Jessica Stone, Ph.D.

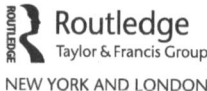
Routledge
Taylor & Francis Group

NEW YORK AND LONDON

First published 2023
by Routledge
605 Third Avenue, New York, NY 10158

and by Routledge
4 Park Square, Milton Park, Abingdon, Oxon, OX14 4RN

*Routledge is an imprint of the Taylor & Francis Group, an
informa business*

© 2023 Jessica Stone

The right of Jessica Stone to be identified as author of this work
has been asserted in accordance with sections 77 and 78 of the
Copyright, Designs and Patents Act 1988.

All rights reserved. No part of this book may be reprinted or
reproduced or utilised in any form or by any electronic,
mechanical, or other means, now known or hereafter invented,
including photocopying and recording, or in any information
storage or retrieval system, without permission in writing from
the publishers.

Trademark notice: Product or corporate names may be
trademarks or registered trademarks, and are used only for
identification and explanation without intent to infringe.

Library of Congress Cataloguing-in-Publication Data
Names: Stone, Jessica (Child psychologist), author.
Title: Technology in mental health : foundations of clinical use /
by Jessica Stone.
Description: First edition. | New York, NY : Routledge, 2023. |
Series: Routledge focus on mental health | Includes
bibliographical references and index. |
Identifiers: LCCN 2022033853 (print) | LCCN 2022033854
(ebook) | ISBN 9780367773595 (hbk) | ISBN 9781032414874
(pbk) | ISBN 9781003171799 (ebk)
Subjects: LCSH: Mental health services--Technological
innovations. | Medical telematics.
Classification: LCC RA790.5 .S757 2023 (print) | LCC RA790.5
(ebook) | DDC 610.285--dc23/eng/20220816
LC record available at https://lccn.loc.gov/2022033853
LC ebook record available at https://lccn.loc.gov/2022033854

ISBN: 978-0-367-77359-5 (hbk)
ISBN: 978-1-032-41487-4 (pbk)
ISBN: 978-1-003-17179-9 (ebk)

DOI: 10.4324/9781003171799

Typeset in Times New Roman
by MPS Limited, Dehradun

Contents

1   Technology in Mental Health: Before,
During, and After COVID-19   1

2   The Slow-to-Warm Approach   6

3   Fundamental Concepts   20

4   Behavioral Neuroscience   49

5   Uses, Standards, and Rights   72

6   Clinical Concepts   86

7   Hardware and Software   97

8   Case Examples   119

9   Fear Less   141

    Index   143

1 Technology in Mental Health: Before, During, and After COVID-19

The use of technology in mental health treatment has forged a winding path. Over multiple decades, a quiet group of professionals, spread throughout the globe, have explored and utilized multiple facets of technology within mental health treatment. Others have eschewed the lure of the new in favor of the traditional. However, over time and as each generation matures, transitions happen and the once new becomes the norm. So, it has been since the beginning of human existence. The new challenges the norm, the new becomes the norm, and a newer-new comes along to challenge the once new, now-norm.

Technology is classically defined by Merriam-Webster as "the practical application of knowledge especially in a particular area", "a capability given by the practical application of knowledge", and "a manner of accomplishing a task especially using technical processes, methods, or knowledge" (Merriam-Webster, 2022, para 2). A deeper search into the meaning of "modern technology" provides the following definition: "methods, systems, and devices which are the result of scientific knowledge being used for practical purposes." (Collins, 2022, para 2).

Colloquially in 2022, technology refers to more 21st century modern advancements, particularly those of a digital nature. Therefore, the use of the word technology in this text is intended to refer to the *practical application of digitally based tools using scientific knowledge in a particular area*. The focus of this book is the use of early 21st century technology within mental health treatment. The first line from Woodworth's *Psychology: A Study of Mental Life* (1921), begins with "Modern psychology is an attempt ..." (p. 1). It is clear that even "modern" is a relative term. Everything is understood within the context of the history, present, and future of knowledge of human beings, with fundamental psychological constructs forming the foundation from which to spring.

DOI: 10.4324/9781003171799-1

COVID-19

As of June 2022, 529,410,287 cumulative cases of Coronavirus (COVID-19) have been reported globally. There have been 6,296,771 cumulative deaths (World Health Organization, 2022). COVID-19 changed lives in what felt like an instant; the loss has been unimaginable with permeations in many directions. Loss and grief have been common threads in the experiences of so many. Two years later, when people are fatigued and hope to return to "normal life", 204,539 cases have been reported (World Health Organization, 2022). It is difficult for many to envision what "normal" would even be at this point.

Prior to COVID-19, the United States had mental health need "rumblings". It was acknowledged that the process to obtain and receive mental health services was less-than-optimal, however, little action seemed to be taken. As of April 2022, Mental Health America reports that over 5.4 million people completed a mental health screening in 2021. This represents a 500% increase in completed screenings in 2019. In 2021, 76% of users in their United States database endorsed items indicating moderate to severe mental health issues between the 2019 and 2021 years. Of these reports, 63% stated loneliness and isolation as one of the top three concerns contributing to their mental health status; 49% endorsed past trauma, and 37% reporting problems within relationships. Screenings for depression and anxiety were the most frequented for 2020 and 2021 (Mental Health America, 2022).

Impact on Mental Health Services

In the initial scramble, clinicians worked to find ways to keep their clients, their families, and themselves safe. Human-to-human contact was discouraged and most mental health sessions moved to primarily online platforms. Many clinicians were thrust into adjustments regarding the way they provided services. This shift included a necessary process of taking inventory of the components involved in the services they have historically provided in an effort to translate the components to an online telemental health platform.

Statistics for 2021 or 2022 are not available at this time, however, 2020 statistics show that the use of and interest in telehealth grew dramatically. Some clients were comfortable with or required telephone sessions, however, many preferred to see and hear each other through a telehealth platform. In the United States, the average increase in telehealth usage of 8335.51%. was found between April 2019 and April 2020 (Fair Health, 2020). The percentage of telehealth usage for the U.S.A. in April 2019 was 0.15% and for April 2020 it was 13.00%. For clinicians, the American Psychological Association (APA) found that 75% of clinicians were exclusively seeing clients remotely in 2020 (Edwards-Ashman, 2021; Stone, 2022).

Initially, many clinicians struggled with the logistics of an online, virtual practice. People wondered: If I (clinician) am freaking out and my life is upside-down, how can I help my clients? What are the legal and ethical requirements within in federal, state, licensing, professional, and malpractice levels? What are the safety concerns/how to I manage safety concerns? What will the impact on rapport be? How will we maintain continuity of care when we are no longer in the same physical space? *What do we actually do?*

The answers to these critical questions predominantly lie in key directives provided by Stone (2022):

1 Apply the fundamental tenets of your training and experience to a new medium – the digital platform. This includes everything from case conceptualization and treatment planning to direct use interventions and collateral contact conversations.
2 Research your legal and ethical requirements and keep records of your findings.
3 Apply such findings from your research to the programs and platforms chosen to provide services in this new medium and document how these choices meet the required criteria you have researched. Vetted resources will need to have been chosen with defined criteria in mind (i.e. HIPAA compliance).
4 Create all the appropriate legal and ethical documents needed, including specific telehealth informed consent.
5 Assess clients for appropriateness for telehealth treatment. This will include safety, diagnostic, access, socio-economic, family dynamics, and cultural considerations.
6 Seek out supervision and/or consultation from industry leaders, just as you would with any new component in your work.

(p. 45–46) *Reprinted with permission.

Since that early spring of 2020, providers have settled into routines within virtual practices, returned to their pre-pandemic in-person, face-to-face sessions, or created a hybrid practice. The American Psychological Association polled U.S. psychologists in 2021 of whom 96% responded that telehealth is therapeutically effective and 97% stated that telehealth services should remain available post-pandemic (Clay, 2022).

Digital Tools Provide Service Expansions

For psychologists, a key to providing telemental services was the expansion of the Psychology Interjurisdictional Compact, or PSYPACT. This compact allows psychologists to provide telehealth services across state lines, as long as they are licensed in good standing in their home state, the home state is included in the PSYPACT legislation, the EPassport requirements are met, and the client is physically in a PSYPACT state. As of June 2022, 33 states had enacted PSYPACT participation and 28 were actively effective. Another five states were in the process toward enactment (PSYPACT, 2021; Clay, 2022). Additionally, the Counseling Compact intends to allow licensed counselors similar license expansion. Eleven states have enacted the legislation and eleven more are in the process of enactment as of June 2022 (Counseling Compact, 2022).

These compacts are much needed advancements in the accessibility of mental health services. Not only can a client receive telemental health services outside of their geographic circle, they can also seek out specialty services depending on their needs. Additionally, military, divorced, and/or estranged families can receive services from the same therapist despite being physically located in different places. People with transportation and/or mobility difficulties can also be seen without the need for travel.

For some practitioners, the use of technology within sessions pre-dated the COVID-19 shifts in the delivery of mental health services. These pioneers were perfectly poised for the inclusion of technology within sessions, and by default, so were their clients. With a few potential adjustments, clinicians and clients alike picked up where they left off and focused on the more broad impacts of the changes in life while using digital platforms and tools.

For others, the swift and somewhat forceful thrust into the use of anything technologically focused within mental health sessions was jarring, overwhelming, and created a sense of chaos that risked undermining the treatment itself. The exploration became multilayered and multifaceted: what are the logistical components and how are they best configured? How do the traditional approaches translate to a digitally based medium? How can the quality of services provided to clients be preserved while exploring relatively unchartered territory?

The impetus for this book lies in these questions and more. Exploring the fundamentals of the incorporation of both telemental health platforms and digital tools in mental health treatment creates a spiderweb of connections and concepts. If we are to understand the ways a concept can be translated into another medium, then we must explore, define, and understand the underpinnings of both the origin and the destination. It is in this that the competency, comfort, congruence, and capability within the use of such therapeutic technology can be achieved (Stone, 2022).

References

Clay, R.A. (2022, January 1). Telehealth proves its worth. *American Psychological Association.* https://www.apa.org/monitor/2022/01/special-telehealth-worth

Collins (2022). *Modern technology.* https://www.collinsdictionary.com/dictionary/english/modern-technology

Counseling Compact (2022). *Counseling compact.* https://counselingcompact.org/map/

Edwards-Ashman, J. (2021, January/February). Advocacy will help secure expanded telehealth coverage. *Monitor on Psychology, 52*(1), 83–85.

Fair Health (2020). Monthly telehealth regional tracker, Apr. 2020. https://s3.amazonaws.com/media2.fairhealth.org/infographic/telehealth/apr-2020-national-telehealth.pdf

Mental Health America (2022). Mental health and COVID-19. https://mhanational.org/mental-health-and-covid-19-two-years-after-pandemic

Merriam-Webster (2022). *Technology.* https://www.merriam-webster.com/dictionary/technology

PSYPACT (2021). *About us.* https://psypact.site-ym.com/page/About

Stone, J. (2022). *Digital play therapy: A clinician's guide to comfort and competence*, 2nd ed. Routledge.

Woodworth, R.S. (1921). *Psychology: A study of mental life.* Henry Holt and Company.

World Health Organization (2022). WHO coronavirus dashboard. *World Health Organization.* https://covid19.who.int/

2   The Slow-To-Warm Approach

Psychology has a long, tumultuous history which is steeped in philosophy, religion, fear, and human nature. To understand therapeutic digital technology, and the slow-to-warm approach toward incorporation to date, it can be helpful to explore the historical underpinnings which tend to linger even in the 21st century. The path to change within the discipline of psychology has been difficult and confusing.

This is not to say that new approaches should be accepted without scrutiny. With a focus on the adage, "do no harm", mental health practitioners want to preserve and protect the therapeutic relationship and integrity of the work. This is a concept to retain throughout time. How then do we evaluate any new approaches for incorporation and use in mental health treatment work?

Exploring the ultimate nature of psychology, therapy, and congruence, along with concepts such as do no harm, soul-mind-body, and ultimately our search for "why", sets the stage regarding the approach to therapeutic digital tool incorporation. Once we understand the slow-to-warm approach, we can address, modify, research, and further shape the incorporation moving forward. How we conceptualize the work itself, the theoretical underpinnings, the client and clinician contributions, and decisions about interventions shapes every aspect of mental health treatment. This also applies to utilizing digital therapeutics: specifically incorporating digital tools in therapy whether that is within telemental health or in-person sessions.

Essence

Essence is the "ultimate nature of a thing" (Merriam Webster, 2021a, para 1). When understanding concepts on a fundamental level, it is important to investigate and recognize the essence of their meaning, tenets, and ultimate nature. Human nature and clinical psychology are

DOI: 10.4324/9781003171799-2

no different. To understand the essence of psychology is to enjoy the freedoms of appropriate implementation and application to the work.

The essence of utilizing digital tools directly in session is the same as any other tool one might employ. This may seem foreign to some, but the underlying therapeutic conceptualizations and goals remain within the incorporation of digital tools. The primary difference is the medium used to convey and communicate within a therapeutic session. If the medium includes the underlying mechanisms for expression, understanding, and change, then the vehicle of the medium matters little.

What and Why

As clinicians, it is imperative that we understand the "what and why" of the work we are doing so that we may remain flexible in our approach. These are our building blocks. From here we can translate skills from one medium to another and meet the needs of our clients. Trends and interests will change over the time of a clinician's career. If the what and why are understood at a core level, then the new *anything* will not be a disruption, rather it will be an avenue to explore. Queries can include: what does this mean to the client? What does the client connect with, or not? How does this complement and/or contribute to the client's life, or not?; and much more.

This brief Routledge focus book intends to provide the reader the fundamentals of utilizing digital technology tools in therapeutic mental health settings. Entering our client's world and gaining insight to their perspectives provides a sense of safety for the client; to be known, heard, seen, and understood – to have importance. These concepts are included in the fundamentals of self-esteem and self-confidence. To have a place; to recognize one's self and one's place in the world leads to understanding self-and-other, connection, stability, and safety. The theme of essence is interwoven.

The Client

Therapy is a joint effort. The client brings their own perspectives, beliefs, experiences, understandings, conceptualizations, history, interpretations, culture, interests, and more. A primary reason a clinician pursues an in-depth intake early in the therapeutic interaction is to understand what the client has experienced, how these experiences have affected them, and to incorporate that information into the case conceptualization and treatment plan. This holistic pursuit brings together the essence of the therapy.

The client is not a passive participant in the therapeutic relationship; rather, the client is an integral partner in the change process. Differing from the historical hierarchical view of the therapeutic relationship, wherein the clinician is the expert and the client/patient is the recipient, a more modern approach is to acknowledge what each contributes to the dyad. This exchange of client perspective and clinical expertise culminates in the therapeutic process and ultimately, shifts will occur.

The Clinician

Just as the client brings a variety of unique aspects into the therapeutic interaction, so does the clinician. The clinician's personal and professional belief systems are present and serve the therapeutic process best when known to the clinician. Awareness allows the clinician to identify what aspect of each might impact the therapeutic process for the client. Personal reflection, therapy, and supervision can assist in identifying what aspects of the clinician's contribution to the therapeutic relationship need further processing and/or boundaries, or could result in the need to give the client a referral. "One size fits all" is not a mantra for therapy.

Person-centered therapy, as addressed by Dr. Carl Rogers, speaks to the importance of "congruence between the actual and ideal self" (Stone, 2022, p. 33; De Lagrave, 2022; Rogers, 1995). The clinician's presentation in session provides the structure and boundaries of the interaction. Rogers advocated for clinicians to remove any existing façades; to focus on being real and genuine. This congruence within the clinician allows the client the freedom and space to achieve self-actualization, grow, and change (Rogers, 1995; Stone, 2022). A clinician's understanding of the fundamental tenets, the hardware, the software, and the relationship provides a solid base for digital therapeutics.

Digital

As stated earlier, trends and interests will change over time and the client who senses a safe environment and secure rapport attachment will want to incorporate such topics into the therapeutic work. Current trends and interests in the 21st century frequently include or incorporate items of a digital nature. This may be of necessity for work, school, and/or the functions of daily life (banking as one example) or it may be for personal reasons (connection, entertainment, etc.).

Day-to-day digital tool use can include the need for connection through messaging programs or social media, whether that be for professional reasons, such as LinkedIn, or for personal reasons, as in Snapchat and Facebook. Connecting to others can lead to business leads and resources, such as opportunities, trainings, and/or research. The world can become a "smaller" place with the ability to connect to people from many different areas. Using digital technology for personal reasons can help people stay in touch, feel much less isolated, and connect with like-minded people/groups. Frequently such connections can lead to a sense of community and inclusion, a goal most humans strive toward. There are two sides to this "coin", and as with anything, there can be pros and cons. However, here we are focused on the impetus and drive behind such use. Time will continue to reveal the balance in our lives regarding digital tools.

Entertainment is another enormous sector within technology. This includes a wide variety of two- and three- dimensional programs, including applications (apps) and games. Self-exploration, identification, practicing social and coping skills, communication, practice, mastery, frustration tolerance, and expression are but a few of the offerings within digital entertainment opportunities. Understanding what your client utilizes and why can be a powerful way to understand them and their day-to-day lives.

Exploring Roots Before Moving Forward

> *Perspectives for the sociology of scientific knowledge are an important reminder not to take for granted the discontinuities between what we are doing now and what has gone before. These distinctions are achieved in the ways we research and write about the new technologies and the ways in which we organize our disciplinary boundaries.*
>
> (Hine, 2005, pp. 6–7)

The History of Traditional Therapies

As stated in the introduction, it is imperative that we explore, define, and understand the underpinnings of both our origin and the destination if we are to translate concepts from one medium to another. As clinicians we have professional and ethical responsibilities to know what we are doing and why we are doing it. To that end, a bit of a deep dive into historical concepts is necessary.

Modern day clinicians (currently defined as the 21st century) have incorporated a number of concepts into their professional work. Some of these have deep roots in the history of humans – philosophy, medicine, and psychology. Some of them are more current concepts which integrate knowledge modern tools have afforded, such as neurobiology. As humans learn more about themselves and the world around them, more and more clarity will be achieved regarding the concepts that need to be retained as fundamental to the human experience, and those which are no longer supported in light of current information. It is not a focus on dismissing the old and adopting the new; it is to think critically about the origins of the fundamentals so they may be analyzed and that which is retained can be appropriately applied to current needs.

"Do No Harm"

A key facet of providing services within a healing profession is the desire to "do no harm". There are two key concepts under this umbrella – Ahimsa and The Hippocratic Oath. Both can be called upon to convey the importance for helping professionals to be intentional in the care provided for others. This powerful concept informs many of the structures and approaches employed with those who are seeking help. One side of this coin is protection: the protection of those seeking help so that they may experience improvements for that which ails them. The other side of the coin can be restriction: that which is different may pose enough of a potential risk that it should not be considered. Both sides of the coin should be explored.

Ahimsa (अहिंसा) (~3rd-century BCD) is a Sanskrit word which derives from *san*, a verb root, and *hims*, with an additional *a* to denote a negation. San means "to kill" and hims means "desirous to kill" and the negating "a" transforms the word into "to be without harm; to be utterly harmless, not only to oneself and others, but to all living beings" (Ponnu, n.d., para. 3). Ahimsa is one of the five yamas, or moral and ethical principles to strive toward. The intention of the word is much more holistic than the direct translation of the word. Ahimsa is a perspective regarding life; it is a way of conceptualizing every aspect of life and impacts our thinking, feeling, moving, and interacting with nature, animals, humans, and more. It is a fundamental benevolence. In the application to health care, Ahimsa can be a holistic way to refer to the concept of "do no harm" we often quote today.

The Hippocratic Oath is a concept that many refer to in the 21st century even though it was written 2,000 years ago (~between the 5th- and 3rd-century BCE). This oath may not be required or integrated formally for mental health practitioners, but the premise remains. This is the basis of education, of certification, and of evidence-based practice. Our clients entrust us with the most delicate information and we work to assist them in ways that will enrich their lives and allow them to move forward. In particular, when a new modality is presented such as utilizing digital technology in direct mental health services, this concept of do not harm is evoked, as is appropriate.

As will become apparent quickly, definitions and fundamental concepts are imperative along this journey. Initially the outline for this text did not include the components of the Hippocratic Oath. It seems to be a document that we are merely aware of; passed down through time, referenced often, and distilled down to the concept of "do no harm". However, the "rabbit hole" of research to find the original source led to a realization that the distilled version is quite different in some ways from the original. The original text does state "I will do no harm or injustice to them", however, this quote focuses on dietary regimens. The original also pledges an allegiance to the "teacher" at a level equal to one's parents and a promise to teach knowledge to the teacher's offspring without any "fee or contract" for those who would want to learn (North, 2002). Yet another example of the purpose for exploring, defining, and understanding as much as is possible so that the foundation from which we spring is solid; not all that is distilled through time is accurate or complete. It is appropriate for concepts to change over time, however, the point is to be aware of the evolution.

Here is a translation of the original Hippocratic Oath (Ορκος) by Michael North of the National Library of Medicine (2002):

> I swear by Apollo the physician, and Asclepius, and Hygieia and Panacea and all the gods and goddesses as my witnesses, that, according to my ability and judgement, I will keep this Oath and this contract:

> To hold him who taught me this art equally dear to me as my parents, to be a partner in life with him, and to fulfill his needs when required; to look upon his offspring as equals to my own siblings, and to teach them this art, if they shall wish to learn it, without fee or contract; and that by the set rules, lectures, and every other mode of instruction, I will impart a knowledge of the art to my own sons, and those of my teachers, and to students bound by this contract and having sworn this Oath to the law of medicine, but to no others.

I will use those dietary regimens which will benefit my patients according to my greatest ability and judgement, and I will do no harm or injustice to them.

I will not give a lethal drug to anyone if I am asked, nor will I advise such a plan; and similarly I will not give a woman a pessary to cause an abortion.

In purity and according to divine law will I carry out my life and my art.

I will not use the knife, even upon those suffering from stones, but I will leave this to those who are trained in this craft.

Into whatever homes I go, I will enter them for the benefit of the sick, avoiding any voluntary act of impropriety or corruption, including the seduction of women or men, whether they are free men or slaves.

Whatever I see or hear in the lives of my patients, whether in connection with my professional practice or not, which ought not to be spoken of outside, I will keep secret, as considering all such things to be private.

So long as I maintain this Oath faithfully and without corruption, may it be granted to me to partake of life fully and the practice of my art, gaining the respect of all men for all time. However, should I transgress this Oath and violate it, may the opposite be my fate.

A more modern version was written by Louis Lasagna in 1964, the Academic Dean of the School of Medicine from Tufts University. Interestingly, this version does not mention the "do not harm" distillation in any form. Hippocratic Oath Modern Version (Lasagna, 1964):

I swear to fulfill, to the best of my ability and judgment, this covenant:

I will respect the hard-won scientific gains of those physicians in whose steps I walk, and gladly share such knowledge as is mine with those who are to follow.

I will apply, for the benefit of the sick, all measures [that] are required, avoiding those twin traps of overtreatment and therapeutic nihilism.

I will remember that there is art to medicine as well as science, and that warmth, sympathy, and understanding may outweigh the surgeon's knife or the chemist's drug.

I will not be ashamed to say "I know not", nor will I fail to call in my colleagues when the skills of another are needed for a patient's recovery.

I will respect the privacy of my patients, for their problems are not disclosed to me that the world may know. Most especially must I tread with care in matters of life and death. If it is given me to save a life, all thanks. But it may also be within my power to take a life; this awesome responsibility must be faced with great humbleness and awareness of my own frailty. Above all, I must not play at God.

I will remember that I do not treat a fever chart, a cancerous growth, but a sick human being, whose illness may affect the person's family and economic stability. My responsibility includes these related problems, if I am to care adequately for the sick.

I will prevent disease whenever I can, for prevention is preferable to cure.

I will remember that I remain a member of society, with special obligations to all my fellow human beings, those sound of mind and body as well as the infirm.

If I do not violate this oath, may I enjoy life and art, respected while I live and remembered with affection thereafter. May I always act so as to preserve the finest traditions of my calling and may I long experience the joy of healing those who seek my help.

The modern version of the Hippocratic Oath is used by a number of medical schools to date (PBS/Nova, 2022). Both versions call for a level of professional humility; to consult others, respect and uphold privacy, and treat the whole of a person, not only their affliction. Neither include the direct concept that has withstood the test of time in the vernacular of the layperson: that medical doctors take an oath to "do no harm".

One of the most interesting components of this exploration of the Hippocratic Oath is to recognize the tendencies for human beings to repeat and retain that which may or may not have been the original words or intention, all the while continuing to misattribute said gem to a particular source. All the more reason to understand origins. The concept of doing no harm is of fundamental importance in the healing services, but it is not something all medical doctors swear to – and it is not from the Hippocratic Oath in the ways it has been portrayed throughout time

The concept of doing no harm while doing good is fundamental. Whether it be Ahimsa or the concepts we understand over time from the Hippocratic Oath, the care for those who seek help is paramount. Perhaps it is time for mental health practitioners to own their own version of these important concepts. Along with traditional approaches to therapeutic services, we certainly want these historical concepts to apply to all direct mental health services, including those of a digital nature.

Deep Diving

A deep dive into the history of psychology, which is essentially a history of humans, yields a plethora of fascinating information. Key people have marked their place in history through the recordings of their beliefs and plights. One of the benefits of reviewing history is the ability of the reviewer to more objectively survey the patterns and paths of those who have lived before, along with how these inform current belief systems. As the reader of this book, one which focuses on the forward movement of psychology and the inclusion of digital tools, you might still wonder what a deep historical dive has to do with the topic at hand. A valid query for certain.

The field of psychology, as a whole, has been slow to change. As a person who has been speaking about, writing about, and utilizing digital tools in therapy for more than a decade, one truth has been revealed many times over: mental health practitioners have a higher level of resistance to that which is new than many other fields. Recent attendance at a conference about virtual reality highlighted these differences. The disciplines of education, medicine, training, and entertainment have all embraced and begun to define their utilization and future plans for virtual, augmented, and mixed reality in their fields. Mental health was the smallest cohort, with fewer speakers and fewer attendees. However, two years ago mental health would not have been included in such a high-profile event ... so there has been a shift. This begs many questions, but a key question for this text is: why is psychology slow to change?

Slow to Warm

Asking this important question brings us back to a review of the history of psychology. It would be rather simplistic to merely place judgment and reduce the field to an encompassing assumption or category. The reality is we have a group of people who have embarked on a career specifically geared toward helping others. Mental health practitioners of all types strive to assist people with that which ails, haunts, plagues, and/or causes them angst. So it cannot be that people in the field are simply steeped so far in tradition that they do not want to change or accept advancements in the field. There must be other reasons for the slow-to-warm approach.

Looking back quite far in history, some patterns certainly emerge. Many of the historical patterns identified regarding the hesitance to change within psychology were fueled by fear – either of individual persecution and/or ridicule, or of unintentionally harming others. Most of the people who disagreed with the beliefs of the time, whichever time period, have not been well regarded. When the tide appeared to turn in a direction other than the prominent status quo of the generation, it would frequently swing back with great force to the more powerful position. This tendency reinforced the reluctance of others to pose any challenge. Historically, people have been killed, ridiculed, shunned, discredited, demoted, and devalued for speaking against the status quo regarding the origins and treatments of mental health concerns.

Philosophy and Psychology

Advanced learning and teaching, as well as psychology, is rooted in philosophy (Merriam Webster, 2021b). A person who earns a traditional doctorate in psychology, for instance, actually earns a doctorate (D.) of philosophy (Ph.), or Ph.D., with a specialty in psychology (more modern times also includes the Psy.D., or doctorate of psychology). There can be variations in the end portion of the person's specializations, but a Ph.D. is a doctorate of philosophy *in something*. This is not to say that a Ph.D. is the only advanced learning in the psychology discipline, rather to highlight the philosophy portion imbedded in the advanced degree.

Philosophy translates to "love of wisdom" (Florida State University, 2021, para 1). "In a broad sense, philosophy is an activity people undertake when they seek to understand fundamental truths about themselves, the world in which they live, and their relationships to the world and to each other" (para 1). One can see how the roots of psychology lie in philosophy. This complex dance has continued throughout human existence.

Psychology stems from early philosophers, or doctors, who pondered questions and taught others, such as Socrates, Plato, and Aristotle (Ahonen, 2019). Each of these three classical ancient Greek philosophers pondered the nature of knowledge toward the logic of argumentation and, ultimately, the scientific method, albeit in different ways. Commonly linked together in their idealism, they had fundamental differences (Woudon, 2021). Socrates (470 BCE–399 BCE), who taught Plato (~428 BCE–348 BCE), had an emphasis in discovering the truth through dialog (McLeod, 2019). Plato, who taught Aristotle (384 BCE–322 BCE), focused on ideal forms and deductive reasoning (McLeod, 2019; aiu, n.d). Aristotle attacked both of his predecessors with his emphasis on logic, empiricism, and induction (McLeod, 2019; aiu, n.d.). Each have informed centuries of philosophical, academic, and ideological pursuits, as well as the formation of psychology.

Psychology is currently defined as the "science or study of the mind and behavior" (Merriam Webster, 2021c, para 1). The word stems from the amalgamation of the Greek words *psychē*, which means "breath, principle of life, life, soul" and *logos*, or "speech, word, reason" (para 3), which has come to be known as -ology, or the study of or branch of knowledge (Lexico, 2022). Psychology has historically been considered the "knowledge of the Soul" (Woodworth, 1921; Merriam Webster, 2021c, para 3). Therefore, people who pursue knowledge in psychology have a love of wisdom regarding the study and knowledge of the soul, mind, and behavior.

Early History

The early history of psychology is steeped in struggles regarding the etiology of mental health difficulties. The separation, or combination, of the mind, soul, and body is central to this struggle. With the approach to care and conceptualization fragmented, people who experienced mental health difficulties were subject to a number of confusing approaches ranging from torture, neglect, and death, to serenity, nurturance, and care. The perceived etiology of the difficulties dictated the treatment.

An Egyptian document called the *Ebers Papyrus* (1550 BCE) was the first known historical mention of clinical depression (Wagner, 2019). The ensuing tumultuous history of philosophical discussions about the mind, body, and soul unfolds after this time, resulting in centuries of confusion. Religion, politics, and power were intertwined in the debate between demonic possessions, supernatural influences, free will, and responsibility, and each have complicated the path to understanding and treatment. There were no firmly agreed upon beliefs about many things within mental health.

This struggle between belief systems that either (1) a God or Gods inflict or relieve humans with/of mental illness or (2) the human body and/or mind was afflicted by something organic spanned an enormous amount of human history. If the person's behavior was due to an affliction of something evil, then attempts to beat, neglect, starve, etc., the demon out of the person would make sense. These attempts would be to free the body and soul from the parasitic usurper. If the behavior was due to a punishment doled out by God or Gods, then the person was being punished by a deity and humans would be better not to challenge that (Graham, 1967). As more information was understood, particularly by physicians such as J.M. Charcot (Owen, 1971), about the human body and the interplay between the body and mind, symptoms could be better understood and therefore treatments could be more properly prescribed.

Lingering

Mental health treatment has historically been perceived as a process which deals with difficulties that were either cast from *within* the person or were cast *upon* the person. This approach is fear-based and highlights the power of the unknown. While most people do not hold these direct views today, a fear-based approach and response to differences has lingered. A human being's tolerance for differences often includes highly revering (if there is perceived value or power, i.e., Shamans of Indigenous Peoples) or to ridiculing that which is frightening or unknown (i.e. judgment, fear).

When we combine the fear of *other,* something that does not readily fit into one's existing paradigm, with a history of fear-based responses, a difficulty with the acceptance of anything new can arise. Just as intergenerational experiences can be passed down throughout time, so can belief systems, particularly if they are incorporated into writings and teachings. History has not always been kind to those who challenge the status quo, therefore a reluctance would be logical to pass forward to future generations.

Change

If we are to promote change and flexibility within psychology, we must recognize that the history has these deep roots in fear, confusion, reverence, and ridicule. Fear and confusion can lead to conservative approaches, particularly with the desire to do no harm. The more we understand these concepts which informed the seminal theories and approaches, the more we can critically approach new developments. The goal is to make decisions to change the historical trajectory, where appropriate, as we become more aware.

References

Ahonen, M. (2019). Ancient philosophers on mental illness. *History of Psychiatry, 30*(1), 3–18. 10.1177/0957154X18803508

aiu (n.d.). *Quantitative research.* https://courses.aiu.edu/QUANTITATIVE%20RESEARCH/2/SEC%202%20QUANTITATIVE%20RESEARCH.pdf#:~:text=reasoning%20by%20Plato%20was%20an%20important%20step%20towards,was%20really%20new%20in%20Parmenides%20was%20his%20axiomatic-

De Lagrave, P. (2022, March 9). The psychology of Carl Rogers: The father of Humanistic psychology. https://www.centerfortheperson.org/the-psychology-of-carl-rogers/

Florida State University (2021). *Department of Philosophy.* https://philosophy.fsu.edu/undergraduate-study/why-philosophy/What-is-Philosophy

Graham, T.F. (1967). *Medieval minds.* George Allen & Unwin Ltd.

Hine, C. (2005). Virtual methods and the sociology of cyber-social-scientific knowledge. In C. Hine (Ed.), *Virtual methods: Issues in social research on the internet,* (pp. 1–16). Berg.

Hippocrates (c. 400 BCE). *Hippocratic Oath (Όρκος).*

Lasagna, L. (1964). *The Hippocratic Oath: Modern version.* Nova/PBS. https://www.pbs.org/wgbh/nova/doctors/oath_modern.html

Lexico (2022). *-ology.* https://www.lexico.com/en/definition/ology

McLeod, S. (2019). *What is psychology?* https://www.simplypsychology.org/whatispsychology.html

Merriam-Webster (2021a). Essence. https://www.merriam-webster.com/dictionary/essence

Merriam Webster (2021b). *The history of "Doctor".* https://www.merriam-webster.com/words-at-play/the-history-of-doctor

Merriam Webster (2021c). *Psychology.* https://www.merriam-webster.com/dictionary/psychology

North, M. (2002). *Greek medicine.* https://www.nlm.nih.gov/hmd/greek/greek_oath.html#:~:text=The%20Hippocratic%20Oath%20%28%20%CE%9F%CF%81%CE%BA%CE%BF%CF%82%29%20is%20perhaps%20the,responsibilities%20similar%20to%20that%20of%20a%20family%20member

Owen, A.R.G. (1971). *Hysteria, hypnosis and healing: The work of J-M Charcot.* Garrett Publications.

PBS/Nova (2022). *The Hippocratic Oath: Modern version.* https://www.pbs.org/wgbh/nova/doctors/oath_modern.html

Ponnu, R. (n.d.). *Ahimsa: Its theory and practice in Gandhism.* https://www.mkgandhi.org/articles/ahimsa-Its-theory-and-practice-in-Gandhism.html

Rogers, C. (1995). *On becoming a person.* Houghton Mifflin Harcourt.

Stone, J. (2022). *Digital play therapy: A clinician's guide to comfort and competence*, 2nd ed. Routledge.

Wagner, B.B. (2019). *The Ebers Papyrus: Medico-magical beliefs and treatments revealed in ancient Egyptian medical text.* https://www.ancient-origins.net/artifacts-ancient-writings/ebers-papyrus-0012333

Woodworth, R.S. (1921). *Psychology: A study of mental life.* Henry Holt and Company.

Woudon, J. (2021). *The similarities between Socrates, Plato, and Aristotle.* Leaf Group Ltd. https://www.theclassroom.com/similarities-between-socrates-plato-aristotle-8698378.html

3   Fundamental Concepts

As suggested in Chapter 2, definitions and fundamental concepts are imperative. To responsibly evaluate anything new for potential inclusion in mental health treatment, we must understand both the fundamentals of the new and the fundamentals of that which we are trying to accomplish – which for our purposes is to provide ethical, responsible mental health treatment while incorporating digital tools.

For example, if we understand the concepts which comprise the concept of connection – if we identify variables which equate to the concept – then we can utilize those variables to evaluate whether or not a concept, tool, or intervention includes or activates connection or, conversely, understand that it does not. We need the identification of such variables and the definitions of each, to identify and evaluate whether or not the variables are part of what we are exploring. Without these, it is a very undefined, amorphous process which can bring us back to the fear-based concepts in Chapter 2.

Some of these concepts are concrete, some are abstract, and some are in progress as we learn more about ourselves and each other. The exploration of abstract concepts is fundamental to being human, however, it is also fraught with complication. Concrete concepts are tangible – i.e., most humans learn that the linguistic representation for a flat surface held up by legs is referred to as a version of "table" in their native language. We can touch that table, measure it, see it, and manipulate it as a concrete item and concept. Scientists and mathematicians can quantify much of what is concrete for abstraction and study.

Abstract concepts depend upon a number of internal and external variables; personal, cultural, societal, etc., and therefore abstract concepts can be difficult to define in terms that others would agree upon. The unknown is that which we explore, extrapolate, and hypothesize until we have more concrete information. From there, we

DOI: 10.4324/9781003171799-3

pursue more knowledge and repeat the processes until we believe we have the proper answers. Even then, some concepts "can be real even though it is not now, or ever, capable of being numerically analyzed" (Siegel, 2012, p. xxviii). That is, until someone comes along in the future with new information and challenges the "standard approaches in the literature", as aptly stated by Borghi et al. (2018).

Beginning This Journey

In the forthcoming pages, you will find a large assortment of inter-twining, often abstract, concepts which impact and inform our *selves,* each other, our experiences in the world, and ultimately, our interactions with our clients in mental health settings. You might wonder why this collection of terms exists in a book about the use of technology in mental health, but, as discussed earlier, understanding and recognizing the fundamentals allows us to apply them to multiple mediums and platforms.

Being

Self, Other, and Self-Other

Self

What is the self and how is it differentiated from other? There are many definitions and ponderings over time. The philosophical quest to understand self is one we will not solve within these pages, but the desire to define it is an important one. When exploring the functions of the brain, interoception, introspection, and the understanding of self becomes central. When we look to self-perception and identification, and therefore representation, the understanding of self is fundamental. Therefore, some time exploring these concepts is well spent.

William James grappled with the concept of self throughout the hundreds of pages within his two-volume book, *The Principles of Psychology* (1918). He attempted to work through the differentiation between being and possession of being, without any concrete conclusion: " ... our bodies themselves, are they simply ours, or are they us?" and "We can see that we are dealing with fluctuating material. The same object being sometimes treated as a part of me, at other times as simply mine, and then again as if I had nothing to do with it at all" (p. 123). William James considered the self to be a representation of one that would be referred to as "me", "myself".

Carl Jung referred to the self as the "total personality" (1971, p. 142), whereas Monti et al. proposed that the "concept of self, i.e. who you think you are, encompasses the sum total of the features that you affirm of your own being and deny of all other beings" (2021, p. 1). What are these features that we might affirm to be of our own being?

In 1954 Kuhn & McPartland attempted to further define and operationalize the self: "The self has been called an image, a conception, a concept, a feeling, an internalization, a self-looking at oneself, and most commonly simply the self (with perhaps the most ambiguous implications of all)" (p.68). In working to create a psychological inventory, Kuhn and McPartland attempted to define the variables and constructs of the self so they might further define what self-meant to people. The inventory was called the Twenty Statements Test and included twenty identical sentence stems, "I am ... ". They categorized the responses to the stems as those of common knowledge (consensual, i.e. consensus; student, daughter, father, etc.) and those needing further explanation (subconsensual, i.e., happy, bored, pretty good at x, etc.) (Kuhn & McPartland, 1954). Overall, the primary categories of responses included physical attributes, social details, roles, group affiliations, and descriptive adjectives.

These were also discussed by Kenny & West (2008), as these authors included social roles, group membership, and interaction partner as the main categories of their self-definition. Furthermore, they explored concepts of self-consistency; to what degree is self-perception consistent across roles? One's self-perception may vary depending of the role, relationship, and interaction and, per the findings of Kenny & West, the consistency of one's self-perception also predicted mental health outcomes (2008). The more consistent the sense of self, the more stable the mental health status; those who perceived themselves as different across a variety of roles reported experiencing more depression, neuroses, and had lower self-esteem. This is also discussed by Festinger (1954) through social comparison theory; our self-perception changes as we compare to ourselves to others.

How we see ourselves, in representation, perception, role, and identity contributes to the realization that we exist as a distinct being from others.

Self-Awareness

Leading us further toward interoception, self-awareness can be traced through a developmental process. Rochat delineated five levels of

Table 3.1 Five Levels of Self-Awareness, Adapted from Rochat, 2003

Level 0: Confusion	The child is unaware of any image or reflection of self as being different from anything else in the environment; the image or reflection is an extension of the existing world. There is no differentiation between self and other.
Level 1: Differentiation	The child is able to perceive that a reflection or picture is different from the surrounding environment; perceptual differentiation; the differentiated self.
Level 2: Situation	Movements in a mirror are explored and recognized as the movements of the self; what is seen in an image or reflection is unique to the self. A situated self is expressed.
Level 3: Identification	The person "manifests recognition" (Rochat, p. 721); the child refers explicitly to themselves when they see their image; the emerging conceptual self; they can refer to the image as themselves.
Level 4: Permanence	The self can be recognized in pictures and movies from the past, where the self might be younger, in unrecognized places, clothing, etc. The permanent self is expressed and represented over time.
Level 5: Self-consciousness	Recognized from a first and third person perspective; aware of both what and how they are in the minds of others.

self-awareness during which a child progresses from Confusion at level 0 to self-consciousness at level 5 (2003). During typical development, a child experiences a process of differentiation between self and other which begins at birth and typically completes between 4 and 5 years of age. The stages include confusion, differentiation, situation, identification, permanence, and self-consciousness (Rochat, 2003); see Table 3.1.

Self-awareness progresses developmentally from confusion to differentiation, situation to identification, permanence to self-consciousness, to lead us toward a recognition of how we may be represented in our minds and the minds of others.

Interoception

Interoception was introduced by C. S. Sherrington in his original 1906 book, *Integrative Action of the Nervous System*, of which originals are difficult to find. Many reprints have been released and the 1947 version allows us a glimpse into the originations of this concept: interoception refers to the physiological sensations which originate from within the body (Sherrington, 1947; Strigo & Craig, 2016). The concept, as many within psychology have, originated within the medical sphere.

A more current redefinition was required as knowledge about the brain has increased dramatically. Chen et al., 2021, define interoception as "the representation of an organism's internal states, and includes the processes by which it senses, interprets, integrates, and regulates signals from within itself" (para 1). Biologically, these sensations which originate physically translate to emotional sensations through the interplay between the autonomic and central nervous systems (Candia-Rivera et al., 2022). This communication, between the central nervous system (CNS) and the autonomic nervous system (ANS) through interoceptive neural circuits, contributes to emotional experiences, the creation of feelings, and decision making (Candia-Rivera et al., 2022; Chen et al., 2021; Fujimoto et al., 2021; Azzalini et al., 2021).

Interoception includes our ability to interpret our internal states of sensing, integrating, and regulating self and emotions through the interplay between the autonomic and central nervous systems, and contributes toward emotional experiences, feelings, and decision making.

Consciousness

Consciousness appears to be interoception's cousin. Another difficult-to-define, abstract enigma, yet common human phenomena, consciousness is an important, yet slippery, concept. Consciousness is, at its simplest, that which is known to us within ourselves. To begin with a classic foundation, we know that Carl Jung discussed the conscious and unconscious in great detail. He discussed consciousness as it is intertwined with the ego:

> *We understand the ego as the complex factor to which all conscious contents are related. It forms, as it were, the centre of the field of consciousness; and, in so far as this comprises the empirical personality, the ego is the subject of all personal acts of consciousness. The relation of a psychic content to the ego forms the criterion of its consciousness, for no content can be conscious unless it is represented to a subject.*
>
> (Jung, 1971, p. 139)

Jung spoke of two experiences of consciousness, the somatic and the psychic. The somatic is similar to what we refer to as interoception; Jung's concept of "endosomatic perceptions" are perceptions that originate from within the body (1971, p. 140). These are not conscious in their entirety, as, per Jung, not all endosomatic stimuli crosses the threshold of consciousness. The psychic is used "only where there is evidence of a will capable of modifying reflex or instinctual processes" (p. 141). Essentially, that which we perceive from the body and that which we understand from the mind falls within the concept of consciousness.

Consciousness, having been represented to the self, includes the known perceptions which originate from within the body and the understandings from the mind.

Introspection

As early as the 1670s, introspection was referred to as a verb to closely examine or inspect something. Deriving from Latin origins, with intro meaning inward and spicere (observe attentively, examine, look at), introspection is not referred to as examining one's own thoughts or feelings until 1807 (Harper, 2022).

At this time, colloquially, introspection refers to "a way of looking inward and examining one's internal thoughts and feelings" (Cherry, 2020, para 4). In looking inward, one is embarking upon the interoceptive process. Sluter, 2015, offers the following about the value of introspection:

1 Introspection *"can be painful because being brutally honest requires us to acknowledge our faults, weakness, failures and shortcomings.*
2 *Examining our own conduct and accepting responsibility for the consequences allows us to move on from mistakes and chart new courses in our relationships.*
3 *Introspection is a gift in that it gives us complete freedom to determine our own future and our own success because we can choose to operate in our areas of strength while acknowledging our weaknesses and managing them.*
4 *Introspection without application of self-knowledge to bring about positive personal change is a wasted opportunity. (Sluter, 2015, para 2)*

Introspection is the mechanism by which we look inward to examine and evaluate our thoughts and feelings.

Perceptions

Perception "walks a line between general and cognitive psychology and philosophical epistemology" (Démuth, 2013). Siegel defines perception as the "process by which external stimuli are received and organized within representations of ongoing experience. Can occur without consciousness but has impacts on internal meaning and external behaviors" (2012, p. A1–59).

Looking more deeply into Siegel's definition, we can conceptualize that something external is being received and organized based on representations, either in an unconscious or conscious matter. These understandings impact how we understand the meaning and therefore our ensuing behaviors. The process within the brain to receive, organize, assign meaning, and then impact behavior is complex and fascinating. Another abstract concept in our chapter, perception has a number of theories associated with its neurological process: bottom-up, top-down, and even a combination approach.

For some, is believed to be a function of the bottom-up approach – starting at the site where external stimuli enters (i.e., the sound waves entering the ear canal and vibrating through the eardrum) and moving upward into more complex portions of the brain through the midline areas of the prefrontal cortex, the precuneus, medial and temporal lobes, lateral and interior parietal cortex, the cingulate cortex, and the default mode network (DMN) (Siegel, 2017). For these theorists, the final perception is determined by the content and quality of sensory input. The sensory input determines the processing of sensory data, and therefore the perception (Démuth, 2013).

When there is a detection of patterns and/or a recognition of stimuli, a top-down approach explains the activation of cortical mappings which are embedded in memories (Siegel, 2017), and these influences are somewhat voluntary. The prior knowledge connects with the stimulus, thereby formulating the perception. Only by understanding the content and "means of mental representation" can cognition, and therefore perceptions, occur (Démuth, 2013, p. 30).

In combination, the higher cortical layers "stream prior knowledge along the same cortical column, even as it takes in the sensory stream from bottom up" (Siegel, 2017, p. 135). Cognitions and memories coming from the top-down, sensory input and memories moving from the bottom up, meet along the cortical column to formulate a more comprehensive cognition. When we understand the constructs of the stimulus (how much of the process is driven my external stimuli), combined with prior knowledge (how much is affected by prior representations), the result is more comprehensive.

These brain structures and their functions will be discussed in the next chapter.

Perceptions combine our prior understandings and experiences with sensory input, observations, and memories to form a more comprehensive cognition.

Theory of Mind

The theory of mind is typically attributed to children as an early developmental stage whereby one becomes able to conceptualize the subjective and internal mental health existence of self and another. Children develop the ability to "detect that another person has a mind with a focus of attention, an intention, and an emotional state" (Siegel, 2012, p. A1–81). This is part of the more comprehensive development of reflective functioning, or the "ability of one person to perceive and reflect upon the mental world of the self and of the other" (p. A1–67).

Frequently credited to Premack and Woodruff's work with chimpanzees, theory of mind encompasses the ability for an individual to impute "mental states to himself and to others (either to conspecifics or to other species as well)" (Premack & Woodruff, 1978, p. 515). If we assume that others experience thinking, believing, wanting, and more, then we can predict the behavior of others, and ourselves, through the anticipation of such experiences. Theory of mind "requires that one can comprehend opaque states in oneself and others" (Leslie, 1987, p. 421).

Theory of mind includes the recognition and anticipation that we and others have internal states; we attempt to attribute qualities to those internal states, and realize that such states may not be clear.

Other

When one is experiencing Rochat's Level 0: Confusion, as described earlier, there is no differentiation of self and other; there is no self-awareness, no boundaries, no distinction. However, when the process begins in Level 1: Differentiation, and works toward Level 5: Self-consciousness, the boundary and distinction between self and other can be perceived and integrated into the knowledge of self.

Perceiving and understanding the sense of other allows for a separation between the thoughts, actions, feelings, experiences, and so much more, which one may distinguish from those of another. Returning again to the ponderings of William James (1918), the self is "fundamentally interpersonal, composed of a repertoire of relational selves" (Kenny & West, 2008, p. 120). However, it is difficult to truly define other, except to say that other is anything that is not self. Self-perception, and therefore other-perception, is relational; conceptualized in relation to self or other. We perceive others once we are able to perceive ourselves, and therefore if it is not ourselves, then it must be other. When we understand the differentiation, on a truly fundamental level, we can then experience empathy, sympathy, and more. If not, we remain in an ego-centric state of "I am hungry, you must be hungry" instead of "I am not hungry, but I understand that you are hungry".

Other can be realized once the self is recognized; the perception and understanding of other allows for a separation from the self.

Self-Other and Double Consciousness

The concept of self-other is one that challenges the binary conceptualization of self and other. Kenny and West postulated that the "relationship between self-perception and perception of others is bi-directional" (2008, p. 134). While the understanding of the boundaries between self and other may be clear, the psychological influence of one toward the other may not be known. The concept of self-other accounts for the psychological relationship and permeable boundaries between the two entities (Schalk, 2011).

Double consciousness was discussed in W.E.B. Du Bois' 1903 book, The Souls of Black Folk. He refers to this experience as: "It is a peculiar sensation, this double-consciousness, this sense of always looking at one's self through the eyes of others, of measuring one's soul by the tape of a world that looks on in amused contempt and pity" (Du Bois, p. 12). The power of this term is palpable and alerts all to a very important concept of looking at one's self through the eyes of others. Not only regarding the realization of another's conceptualization of us, but the comparison of one's self-knowledge to this other's knowledge and the impact on one's self.

Self-other recognizes that the relationship between self and other is bidirectional, with the psychological influence toward each potentially unknown, but accounted for. Double consciousness addresses the concept of looking at one's self through the eyes of others, with a comparison of self-concept and other's-concept, and acknowledgment of the potential impact of all.

In-Group Identification and Relational Selves

In-group identification refers to the ways we understand the self within a group dynamic. How do the ways we self-identify change when we operate within a group dynamic? Research on optimal distinctiveness theory by Brewer (1991) revealed that humans tend to strive toward a "middle ground between group identity and individuality" (p. 475) when in a group. This raises questions about the sense(s) of self, the level of stability required for positive mental health, and the types of variability which are acceptable to remain within a range of optimal functioning.

These queries include the concept of relational selves: "self-perceptions are linked to representations of significant others, and these linkages form specific relational selves for each significant other" (Kenny & West, 2008, p. 121). These are the "aspects of the self-associated with one's relationships with significant others" (Chen et al., 2011, p. 149). Although a stable sense of self can equate to positive mental health status, humans also exhibit relational selves which vary depending on the situation and value of the relationship. Additionally, when speaking of relationships, are people more inclined to strive toward the middle ground because they are attracted to like-minded people? Or are they like-minded people because the members strove toward a middle ground? We can see how humans have grappled with these concepts throughout time.

In-group identification refers to the ways we self-identify within a group dynamic and whether or not the self-identification is stable or variable depending upon the environment. Relational selves include the varied representation of self as it is dependent upon the relationships with others and the potential mental health impacts of a self-identity which has greater variability.

Body

*Brain**

Per Daniel Siegel, the brain is an "extensively distributed set of neurons we call the 'nervous system' and its many components that are interwoven with the body as a whole" (2012, p. xxi).

The brain is a complex, three-pound organ which houses important roles such as: "intelligence, interpreter of the senses, initiator of body movement, and controller of behavior". (NIH, 2022, para 1).

*The purpose of the discussion of the brain here is to distinguish it from the mind; further discussion of the brain structure and functions will be presented in the next chapter.

The brain is a complex organ with an extensive nervous systems and functions.

Mind

The mind is an abstract concept, one that is defined differently by many, including the multidisciplinary professionals consulted by Siegel in his 2012 book, *Interpersonal Neurobiology*. Various disciplines have registered beliefs about the mind: the anthropologist believed the mind is "what is shared across the generations"; the neuroscientist, "the mind is simply the activity of the brain"; the psychologist, "the mind is composed of thoughts and feelings and includes our consciousness and the subjective nature of our internal lives as well as the output of the mind, which are our behaviors" (p. xxi). Siegel proposes that "A core aspect of the mind can be defined as an embodied and relational process that regulates the flow of energy and information" (p. xxvi). "The mind is process and action (or the conscious outcome of process and action), the brain is the mechanism in which that action occurs. While the brain can exist without the mind, the converse is certainly not true" (Uttal, 1987, p. 672).

Relating to our inner and subjective experience, the mind includes being conscious or aware. The mind's information and the flow of energy within our bodies and relationships contributes to our emotion, thinking, and memory. The mind is interdependent with the subjective experiences, awareness, information, consciousness, and relationships within and/or regarding the body. The mind has the power to change the structure of the brain (Siegel, 2012).

Regulating the flow of energy and information, the mind includes being conscious and aware, experiencing emotion, thinking, and memories, and is interdependent with subjective experiences, information, and relationships which impact the body and potentially the structure of the brain.

Neuroplasticity

Neuroplasticity, or brain plasticity, is the term used to discuss the brain's ability to adapt and change in response to a variety of experiences (Cherry, 2022). The brain has the ability to change due to both positive and negative experiences, medical concerns and/or damage, and degenerative disease. Understanding that the brain can change allows treatments to be borne which focus on the health of the brain and ability for change for good. For this reason we will go into some detail regarding neuroplasticity.

The term plasticity was originated by William James, 1890, however, he was referring to behavioral change. He recognized that humans are capable of meaningful change (James, 1918; Cotman & Berchtold, 2002). Therefore, at the time, plasticity referred primarily to behavior. It would take some time for clinicians to adopt positive understandings of neural plasticity.

Early clinicians believed that neurogenesis, the process whereby new neurons are created, ceased after birth; there was no new growth, therefore no plasticity. It was a fixed system. This concept of plasticity was not broadened and applied to the brain until it was found that the structure of the brain can and will change over time. These changes include those of the system, cellular, and molecular levels (Cotman & Berchtold, 2002).

Two early researchers, Ioan Minea and Santiago Ramón y Cajal, attempted to dispute the historical belief that the brain was a non-renewable organ. In the late 1800's and early 1900's, some clinicians believed that plasticity existed in the peripheral nervous system (PNS), but not the central nervous system (CNS) (Stahnisch & Nitsch, 2002). Even psychology's own Sigmund Freud contributed in this arena briefly in the 1880's, having demonstrated neurofibrils between the nerve cell body and its axon within lamprey and crayfish (Illis, 2012).

Despite having received the Nobel Prize in 1906 for the discovery of the neuron, scientists of the time did not believe in Ramón y Cajal's ~1913 theories regarding the plasticity of the central nervous system (Britannica, 2022; Illis, 2012). Neuronal changes he referred to were considered "sprouting", which was deemed pathological in the early 1900's. The acceptance of neural plasticity really did not happen until 1948, when Polish neuroscientist Jerzy Konorski published his discovery of the brain's ability to change (Konorski, 1948; Ossowska, 2021). Additionally, Armstrong et al. demonstrated that the brain of a cat had 15–30,000 boutons termineaux (the end of the axon which connects to other nerve cells) through staining synaptic vesicles (Armstrong et al., 1956; Farlex, 2022a). From this discovery, it was seen that sprouting must have a regenerative quality, not a purely pathological one; new neural branches must be created past infancy.

Although it is possible that neural and psychiatric pathology can be a result of neuroplasticity, the ability for positive change is important to understand (Innocenti, 2022). The long process to understand the ability for the brain to adapt and/or change is another way our conceptualization of treatments and interventions are informed by history. Certainly advancements in technologies made the adoption more palatable, but the long-held, historical adherence to the belief of a fixed state of the brain and the inability for adaptation has influenced our field.

Neuroplasticity is currently conceptualized into two primary categories: functional and structural. Functional neuroplasticity refers to the brain's ability to move a function from one area of the brain to another if the original area is damaged. Structural plasticity includes the brain's ability to change the physical structure due to learning and/or experience.

Over the lifespan we have a variable number of neurons, neuronal sprouting, neuronal regeneration, and neuronal death. By the age of three it is estimated that the human brain has 15,000 synapses per neuron in the cerebral cortex. However, due to synaptic pruning, adults function with approximately half that amount. The neurons we use frequently are strengthened and develop stronger connections. Conversely, the ones we do not use will eventually die (Cherry, 2022). Through these new and strengthened connections and synaptic pruning, the brain is able to maintain its adaptability and plasticity. The more we understand about this process and these abilities, the better informed our interventions and treatments can be.

Neuroplasticity refers to the brain's ability to adapt in both functional and structural ways, with much to learn and enormous implications for psychological treatment, interventions, and understandings.

Cognition and Metacognition

Thinking (cognition) and thinking about thinking (metacognition) are enormous, abstract concepts. Neither the general concepts nor the complex neurobiological processes for either can be sufficiently addressed here, but we will introduce a few fundamental topics to contribute to our discussion. Frontal lobe processes which connect to the amygdala, thalamus, hypothalamus, default mode network (DMN), task positive network (TPN), and so much more are involved in both cognition and metacognition, to varying degrees, and will be important for concept introductions later in the chapter and book.

"'Cognition' is all the mental processes involved in any act or process of acquiring knowledge, including perception, memory, attention, language, thinking, problem-solving and decision-making" (Harappa Diaries, 2021, para 3). We have information and sensations inputted into the body, processed by the brain, and connected with emotions and memories which result in thoughts, and at times, actions. Through clustering and organizing concepts (schemata) and utilizing re-presentations of concepts (prototypes), cognition allows us to strive toward understanding both our internal and external experiences (PressBooks, n.d.).

Metacognition seems to be a bit of an abstract concept squared (Ab^2). It requires abstract thinking about abstract thinking. Metacognition has been defined as "one's thoughts and feelings about acquiring new knowledge" (Harappa Diaries, 2021, para 3). When we think about our own thoughts and feelings, and about the acquisition of new knowledge and cognitions, we can work toward recognition of our own perspectives and apply these understandings to both self-reflective introspective and interoceptive processes. Grounded in perception and action, metacognition defers to various language, social aspects, interoception, and introspection for meaning (Shea, 2018). We use these references to formulate our metacognitions and give them structure.

Cognition and metacognition are enormous, abstract concepts which engage multiple brain structures to process information and sensations, connect them with emotions and memories, and can result in thoughts and/or actions. Cognition can be thought of as thinking, and metacognition as thinking about thinking.

Philosophy and Existentialism

Purpose and Intention

Purpose can be defined as "the reason for which something exists" (Dictionary, 2022a). If the existential question is "Why do we exist?", then "purpose" may well be the answer. An exploration by Ciliberti (2022), reveals that purpose "originates from internal reality ... inside oneself" (para 4). This internal reality, one defined by the self, may be common for humankind: "One wishes to make a good life for oneself, improve oneself, understand reality and find happiness and meaning" (para 4). Happiness and meaning are quite subjective. The seeker of purpose might strive to "find a lifestyle that offers common necessities, pleasure and security, limits pain and unease, optimizes a reduction in my imperfections, offers the opportunity to make sense of my surroundings and the world, and enables a state of sustained meaningful *Eudaimonia*" (para 4).

Eudaimonia is a Greek word translating to happiness, however, it dives into virtues and ethics; purpose. Deriving from Aristotle's Nicomachean Ethics (*Ēthika Nikomacheia*), the concept of Eudaimonia explores the science of happiness (Aristotle, ~335 BCE; Moore, 2019) For Aristotle, the aim toward happiness, is to "identify the good, or happiness, with pleasure; which is the reason why they love the life of enjoyment" (Aristotle, ~335 BCE 1.5, para 8).

Intention can be defined as "a determination to act in a certain way" (Merriam-Webster, 2022a, para 2); "an aim or purpose" (Couch, 2015, para 5). Furthermore, this concept can be separated into future-directed and present-directed intentions, with the former focused more on planning and the latter focused more on producing behavior (Cohen & Levesque, 1990).

Purpose and intention together drive humans toward meaning and reason in a determined way. In psychology, understanding the purpose and intention of the client is imperative when guiding them toward healing. Assigning therapeutic direction which is congruent with one's purpose and intention, planning and behavior, allows for an alignment of meaning within the therapeutic process.

Purpose is the reason something exists; intention is an aim or purpose which serves as determination to act. Together, purpose and intention drive us toward meaningful behavior, planning, and understanding toward meaning and reason.

Existence and Reality

Each of these three subjects: existence, reality, and presence, pose ontological quandaries; they relate to the concept of being. If we can conceptualize aspects of the states of being, then we may be able to identify these within therapeutic interactions. Therefore, the questions become "what are they and what do they mean to us?"

That which exists is an entity. Entities exist as they have an objective reality and a positive existence which is provided by substance. In other words, the entity is made of something and can be objectively perceived, therefore it exists. Such existence can have two levels: 1) existence which does not depend on others; the entity can exist independently and 2) existence which depends on others; they are dependent on other entities which exist and allow others to exist (Varghese, 2018).

In addition, entities can be separated into two forms as well: 1) real entities and 2) functional entities. Real entities exist in space as evidenced by their substance, form and structure; they exist due to their substance. They can act on others and be acted upon. They "have volumetric existence in three-dimensional spatial system" (Varghese, 2018, p. 1). Functional entities lack substance and objective reality, rather, they "exist only in the minds of rational beings and in mathematical analyses" (Varghese, 2018, p. 1). They perform their assigned functions and exist only through the creators. This will become an interesting concept later in the book.

In 1892 David Ritchie wrote an article entitled, "What is reality?". He pondered the internal, psychic experience of reality – that "real is whatever is truly in anyone's experience and is not falsely alleged to be" (Ritchie, 1892, p. 265). The complication becomes apparent when considering the temporary, "subjective reality" of something which is internal and psychic, as opposed to the "objective reality" of real events (Ritchie, 1892, p. 266). Referring back to entities, subjective reality can be likened to functional entities and objective reality to real entities; one exists due to substance, and the other due to the creator.

Ultimately, what is real? If it is a subjective experience, is it not perceived as real to the person? In Ritchie's initial ponderings, that which is in one's experience is real. Then it becomes a distinction between reality for one versus the reality for another, and whether or not we have individualistic or collective realities, or both. Perhaps reality is partially dependent on the impact of the perception either for the individual or the collective, or both.

That which exists has substance and can be objectively perceived, whether they are independent or dependent, real or functional. Reality can be in the 'eye of the beholder'; of subjective or objective qualities to exist due to substance or a creator, and dependent upon perception.

Presence and Telepresence

Presence is referred to as the experience of 'being there'; telepresence is 'being there' in a virtual environment. It is an "a psychological state or subjective perception in which even though part or all of an individual's current experience is generated by and/or filtered through human-made technology, part or all of the individual's perception fails to accurately acknowledge the role of the technology in the experience" (International Society for Presence Research, n.d., para 3). A powerful article by Jonathan Steuer in 1992 explored a variety of concepts associated with telepresence, or the "real or simulated environment in which a perceiver experiences telepresence" (p. 7). The presence in this definition of telepresence is medium-induced.

The term has undergone an evolution over time, from remote manipulation of physical objects, or teleoperations, (Minsky, 1980), to a combination of teleoperations along with the experience within virtual environments (Held & Durlach, 1992). Minsky stated, "telepresence emphasizes the importance of high-quality sensory feedback and suggests future instruments that will feel and work so much like our own hands that we won't notice any significant difference" (1980, para 4). Held and Durlach questioned the limitations of Minsky's definition and posed that telepresence should include "systems that are designed to transform" and is "likely to be useful in a variety of other applications, more specifically, it should enhance performance in applications (i.e. virtual environments) where the operator interacts with synthetic worlds created by computer simulation" (p. 109). As technology has advanced, so has the definition.

Presence and telepresence are distinguished primarily by the environment; both are psychological states or subjective perceptions, however, one is in the physical presence and one is generated by or filtered through human-made technology.

Proprioception

Colloquially, proprioception is body awareness; the ability to conceptualize and navigate the body within an environment and space. Medically, proprioception is a sense of positioning and movement which is mediated by proprioceptors (mechanosensory neurons which convey information about the "stretch and tension of muscles, tendons, and joints") (Vega & Cobo, 2021, p. 1). These neurons supply sensations of heat, cold, and pain to sensory organs in the muscles and tendons. This proprioceptor information travels to the central nervous system through the spinal cord, cerebellum, and the cerebral cortex to be processed (Vega & Cobo, 2021). Further, "Proprioceptive information informs us about the contractile state and movement of muscles, about muscle force, heaviness, stiffness, viscosity and effort and, thus, is required for any coordinated movement, normal gait and for the maintenance of a stable posture" (Kröger & Watkins, 2021, p. 1)

Proprioception allows us to navigate through a variety of environments and spaces via a biological process whereby information is relayed throughout the body and processed by the brain for coordinated movement, gait, and posture.

Embodiment

To embody is to "give a bodily form to; incarnate; to represent in bodily or material form; to make part of a system or whole; incorporate" (Farlex, 2022b, para 1). Embodiment is the experience of being present in our own bodies, or in another through representative means. It is to accept and experience the perception of self, distinct from other, within the representational form. Traditionally, this refers to one's physical body as the body is ever-present (James, 1918). However, the more modern concept of embodiment and its exploration have yielded a more complex nest of possibilities. The rubber hand illusion experiment, whereby a prosthetic hand was stimulated within the sight of the person while the physical hand was simultaneously stimulated, created a belief in the person that the prosthetic was indeed their physical hand, so much so that a hammer strike of the prosthetic caused great fear in the person (Botvinick & Cohen, 1998).

Longo et al., 2008, recreated the rubber hand illusion study with the purpose of expanding and operationalizing the understandings of embodiment. There were able to demonstrate that the "experience of one's own body is not a single dimension, but a composite of several different subjective components organised with a character structure" (Longo et al., 2008, p. 993). With a complex interplay between both top-down and bottom-up influences, it was found that both the immediate sensations and the body's stored representations influenced the embodiment perceptions (Longo et al., 2008).

Being present in a representative form is a complex process. Intertwined with the concepts of self and other, interoception, perception, and even proprioception, embodiment includes the form which we inhabit and of which we claim ownership, either fundamentally or temporarily.

The conceptualization of embodiment is a complex, abstract construct intertwined with self-concept and -perception, whereby the immediate sensations and stored representations influence one's embodiment perceptions.

Experience

Play

Play is considered a "non-instrumental activity", that is, it's purpose and goal is of enjoyment (Weisberg, 2015, p. 249). Play occurs throughout the lifespan (Kaduson, 2015). We certainly identify play as a child's pursuit, however, it is important to acknowledge that play is an important part of life throughout the years.

Weisberg posed that play "encompasses a large range of behaviors that occur throughout the lifespan, including gaming, physical play, word play, construction play, and so on" (2015, p. 250). Children's play often includes physical, cognitive, and social spontaneity, and it creates joy and a sense of humor (Lieberman, 1965). For adults, Schaefer listed five key factors of playfulness in a 28 item scale for adults: fun loving, sense of humor, enjoys silliness, informal, and whimsical (1997). Csikszentmihalyi explored adult reasons for enjoyment. They were either intrinsic, the use of skills and enjoyment of an experience, or extrinsic, competition, prestige, glamor, regard (1990). "The main reasons for devoting time and effort to playing ... are that the experiences are rewarding in themselves, and that the activities provide little worlds of their own which are enjoyable" (p. 14).

Play can be engaging, soothing, expressive, creative, symbolic, pretend, representative, explorative, educational, projective, allow for trial and error, demonstrate cause and effect, and yes, even therapeutic. Identification of the expressed or demonstrated components of play, incorporated with a solid therapeutic foundation, can allow a mental health clinician a view into the window of a client's world, no matter what the age.

Play is a critical component of human nature and development across the lifespan; identification of the expressed or demonstrated components of play allows a view into the world of the player, through the demonstration of enjoyable little worlds.

Pretence and Quarantining

The word "pretence" often conjures up negative connotations, as in "false pretence". However, technically, the definition includes "pretending or feigning; make-believe" (Dictionary.com, 2022b, para 1). Pretending and make-believe are critical components of healthy development. Pretending can blur the lines of self and other, of dictated function, of reality; the act conjures a symbolic understanding and a distinction from reality. The meta-representational and mentalistic qualities of pretending helps us to develop theory of mind (Leslie, 1987; Weisberg, 2015).

Leslie posits that pretence, or the ability to pretend, is the beginning development of the "ability to understand cognition itself" (1987, p. 416), that "we deliberately distort reality". (p. 412). Furthermore, "pretend is a special case of acting as if where the pretender correctly perceives the actual situation", but reality is suspended while engaging in the play (p. 413).

With the prevalence of COVID19, quarantining certainly means something very specific, however, Leslie introduces the concept in relation to pretend play and representation (1987). "Pretense affects the normal reference, truth, and existence relations of the representations it uses" (Leslie, 1987, p. 415). Any primary representational system affected would quickly be undermined by arbitrary meaning changed. To prevent primary representational systems from being affected – and thereby undermining the assigned meaning – "pretend representations must somehow be marked off, or 'quarantined', from primary representations" (Leslie, 1987, p. 415).

It has been demonstrated that children "quarantine appropriately and separate pretense* from reality" (*UK spelling) (Weisberg, 2015, p. 255). Children do not believe "that what has happened in a pretend episode affects how things work in the real world", i.e., quarantining (p. 251.) She explains further,

> *In order to pretend productively and without confusion, children should understand that there is a boundary between pretense and reality. If children truly did not realize that pretend scenarios are separate from reality, as Piaget feared, they would risk blurring what is true in the pretend world with what is true in the real world, and would potentially end up with lots of false ideas about reality. A failure to maintain a strict boundary between pretense and reality could lead to a failure to believe that pretend stipulations are true only in the pretend world, not in reality.*
>
> (Weisberg, 2015, p. 255; Piaget, 1962)

Both pretence and quarantining are important components of play; the ability to employ representational, meta-representational, mentalistic, cognitive, and theory of mind concepts to play, while maintaining the ability to quarantine, allows for free play assignment, expression, and creation.

Experience and Immersion

Experience encompasses a variety of difficult-to-condense components. Merriam-Webster provides the following definitions:

1 direct observation of or participation in events as a basis of knowledge

 a the fact or state of having been affected by or gained knowledge through direct observation or participation

2 practical knowledge, skill, or practice derived from direct observation of or participation in events or in a particular activity
3 something personally encountered, undergone, or lived through
4 the conscious events that make up an individual life

    a   the events that make up the conscious past of a community or nation or humankind generally

5   the act or process of directly perceiving events or reality (Merriam-Webster, 2022b, para 1)

Whether it be observation, participation, knowledge or skill, an encounter, the events that make up our lives, or a direct perception of events or reality, experience is another abstract concept which is a part of all our lives. Bailenson offers the following about experience: "We value it because we know that firsthand exposure to facts or events is the most powerful and effective way for us to learn and understand the world" (2018, p. 5).

Immersion is defined as an "absorbing involvement"; to immerse is to "plunge into something that surrounds or covers especially; to engross" (Merriam-Webster, 2022c). To engross is to "take or engage the whole attention of: occupy completely" (Merriam-Webster, 2022d). The definitions of many concepts in this chapter are multilayered and take a level of commitment to discover the intended essence. To be immersed, based on this exploration, is to be engaged and occupied by an absorptive involvement in or with an experience.

The experience of immersion is described by Csikszentmihalyi as a state of flow, or as defined by flow theory, "the state in which people are so involved in an activity that nothing else seems to matter; the experience itself is so enjoyable that people will do it even at great cost, for the sheer sake of doing it" (1990, p. 4). Immersion can be delineated into a number of categories/types, including: cultural, language, tactile, strategic, narrative, and virtual reality (Crossman, 2018; Beal, 2007).

Experiences populate our memories, inform our cognitions and decision making; they are the building blocks which construct many aspects of who we might become, who we are, and how we move through our lives. Immersion is an engagement within an absorptive, flow-like state and experience.

Immersive experiences can transcend the physical reality, whether internally or externally, dependent upon the environment and stimuli, to create an absorptive experience.

Relationship, Connection, and Community

A relationship is the way in which two (or more) things are connected (Cambridge Dictionary, 2022). Relationships and connection with others are central to health and well-being of our body, mind, and soul.

Feeling heard, seen, understood, and accepted with a relationship can alleviate loneliness, provide us with purpose, and propel us to strive for more (Perun, 2022). We are fueled by relationships, whether they be friends, family, romantic, business, or any other type imaginable.

According to Cushman and Cahn Jr, interpersonal relationships can be understood through four primary perspectives: social rules, symbolic interactionist, action theory, and systems (1985). These are but a small sampling of the possible perspectives, however, one can see that relationships are complex and cannot be deemed mutually exclusive from a number of human experiences. Please refer to Table 3.2 for clarification. Relationships, connection, and community are all intertwining concepts within our chapter's exploration; self, other, self-other, double consciousness, in-group identification, and theory of mind are all important concepts within.

The sender, receiver, message, and interpretation of meaning are central components of communication. Verbal or non-verbal messages and feedback are exchanged between the sender and receiver, and the context, environment, history, and nature of the relationship will all impact the communication (Nordquist, 2019).

Communication is a central component of relationships forming, developing, maintaining, and terminating. As stated, communication can be verbal or non-verbal and is utilized to convey thoughts

Table 3.2 Four Interpersonal Relationship Perspectives, adapted from "Communication in Interpersonal Relationships", by D.P. Cushman & D.D. Cahn, 1985, SUNY Press

Perspective	Description
Social Rules	establishing, maintaining, and terminating interpersonal relationships are (1) guided and governed by socially established rules (2) occurs through communication (3) share a common code and interactional system
Symbolic Interactionist	our self-concept, is a symbolic creation formed and sustained in our interaction with others; we must communicate and sustain our identity in our interactions with others; the recognition of our identity by others gives reality to the self
Action Theory	our interpersonal relationships are constructed out of different types of reciprocal self-concept support
Systems	our self-concept, and in turn our interpersonal relationships, are significantly influenced by our participation in organizational, cultural, and cross cultural interactional systems

and feelings and to connect with others. James Carey defined communication as "a symbolic process whereby reality is produced, maintained, repaired and transformed" (2009, p. 19). He further explained that

> communication through symbolic and other forms, comprises the ambience of human existence. The activities we collectively call communication – having conversations, giving instructions, imparting knowledge, sharing significant ideas, seeking information, entertaining and being entertained – are so ordinary and mundane that it is difficult for them to arrest our attention.
>
> (Carey, 2009, p. 19)

His point being, that communication can become so wrote and expected that we can miss the importance, the nuances, the messages, the wonderment ...

The word community conjures positive feelings of belonging and acceptance for many. Community is both a feeling and a set of relationships among people which impacts our health and well-being (Chavis & Lee, 2015). People form and maintain communities to meet common needs. Chavis and Lee explain that "Members of a community have a sense of trust, belonging, safety, and caring for each other. They have an individual and collective sense that they can, as part of that community, influence their environments and each other" (2015, paras 4–5). Humans experience many different communities within any given day.

Communities "allow people to interact with each other, share experiences, develop valued relationships and work toward a common goal" (Reference, 2020). Positive communities foster growth, development, connection, relationships, support, and self-worth for people of all ages. Like-minded people who share common interests and goals tend to connect within communities. Modern technologies advancements such as the phone, internet, and video communication platforms have created opportunities for communities to come together in expansive ways and can lead to stronger connections which result in increased community-belonging benefits.

Through a variety of environments and perspectives, relationships bring two or more people together to form connections, and hopefully a community, so the participants can benefit in ways that impact all parties; how people see themselves, each other, and their worlds have reciprocal impacts on the health and well-being of all participants.

Identification and Representation

Building upon the concepts within this chapter, identification, representation, and thereby recognition, continue the intertwining process. What it means to the self and others, and the multi-dimensional impacts of each, to identify and represent in congruent manners – and to be recognized for such – propels our existence to levels of profound magnitudes.

Identification, or self-identification, revolves around many of the concepts presented in earlier sections, and deserves independent recognition as well. As we develop, the way we see ourselves in the world impacts our emotions, relationships, connections, community, decision making, trajectories, and our physical bodies. The congruence of owning and accepting our true and identified self provides a level of peace and tranquility; a fundamental truth.

Much of the analytic therapeutic experience can be simplified to a process by which we pursue the true self. This true self does not exist in a vacuum; it impacts and is impacted by relationships and the environment. However, true knowledge, acceptance, and congruency of self breeds an enviable high quality of communication and relationships. This pursuit is lifelong, like that of Saddartha. The process toward self-actualization (fulfillment and development of one's abilities and appreciation for life, [Maslow, 1943; Perera, 2020]) is worthy even if the ultimate goal is not ultimately realized.

There are many aspects of representation; we return to the concepts of self and other. How one identifies the important aspects of their own representation – to themselves and to others … How others recognize (or don't), accept (or don't), respect (or don't) one's self – or community representation impacts our identity within ourselves and with others; in our own minds and in the minds of others.

Our minds, bodies, and souls can be vulnerable to society's response to our identities and representation. Representation of our true self-identification holds immense power and it is vital to recognize and honor it, particularly as mental health clinicians. Color, culture, religion, nationality, interests, gender identity, sexual identity, language, appearance, and beliefs are but a few of the different representations important to human beings.

Mis-representation can deteriorate one's self-identification; it can deafen the important voice of many.

Recognition by self and others of one's identity and representation can fulfill (at least in part) the fundamental need to be seen, heard, accepted, and understood. Appropriate recognition can have elements of inclusivity; to be recognized for the components of self-identification and representation can result in knowing (self and others). There is power in knowing.

Identification and representation of the self to ourselves and others impacts how we feel about ourselves, the world, and our place within it; to honor and respect one's self can lead to truth and knowing; self-acceptance and identity; purposeful steps toward self-actualization.

This journey of foundation has been tremendous. Presenting such concepts comprehensively within a few pages lends itself to summaries when volumes could be (and have been) written about each. Philosophers, educators, researchers, and clinicians alike have pondered these concepts for generations, and will most likely continue to do so.

May we continue to grow, change, adapt, and incorporate knowledge and understandings along the way so that we as a species can move toward actualization. Only then will we truly honor ourselves and one another.

References

Aristotle (~335 BCE). *Nicomachean ethics.* http://classics.mit.edu/Aristotle/nicomachaen.mb.txt

Armstrong, J., Richardson, K.C., & Young, J.Z. (1956). Staining neural end feet and mitochondria after post-chroming and carbowax embedding. *Stain Technology, 31,* 263–270. https://www.tandfonline.com/doi/abs/10.3109/10520295609113816

Azzalini, D., Buot, A., Palminteri, S., & Tallon-Baudry, C. (2021). Responses to heartbeats in ventromedial prefrontal cortex contribute to subjective preference-based decisions. *Journal of Neuroscience, 41*(23), 5102–5114.

Bailenson, J. (2018). *Experience on demand: What virtual reality us, how it works, and what it can do.* Norton.

Beal, V. (2007). Immersion. *Webopedia.* https://www.webopedia.com/definitions/immersion/#:~:text=Immersion%20is%20the%20act%20of%20fully%20submerging%20something,in%20this%20context%20when%20referring%20to%20video%20games

Borghi, A.M., Barca, L., Binkofki, F., & Tummolini, L. (2018). Varieties of abstract concepts: Development, use and representation in the brain. *Philosophical Transactions of the Royal Society B: Biological Sciences, 373.* https://royalsocietypublishing.org/doi/pdf/10.1098/rstb.2017.0121

Botvinick, M. & Cohen, J.D. (1998). Rubber hand "feels" what eyes see. *Nature, 391,* 756. https://www.nature.com/articles/35784.pdf

Brewer, M.B. (1991). The social self: On being the same and different at the same time. *Personality & Social Psychology Bulletin, 17*(5), 475–482.

Britannica (2022). Santiago Ramón y Cajal. *Encyclopaedia Britannica.* https://www.britannica.com/biography/Santiago-Ramon-y-Cajal

Cambridge Dictionary (2022). Relationship. *Cambridge Dictionary*. https://dictionary.cambridge.org/dictionary/english/relationship

Candia-Rivera, D., Catrambone, V., Thayer, J.F., Gentili, C., & Valenza, G. (2022). Cardiac sympathetic-vagal activity initiates a functional brain-body response to emotional arousal. *PNAS, 119*(21). https://www.pnas.org/doi/10.1073/pnas.2119599119

Carey, J. (2009). *Communication as culture: Essays on media and society, revised*. Routledge.

Chavis, D.M. & Lee, K. (2015, May 12). What is community anyway? *Stanford Social Innovation Review*. https://ssir.org/articles/entry/what_is_community_anyway

Chen, S., Boucher, H., & Kraus, M.W. (2011). The relational self. In S.J. Schwarz, K. Luyckx, & V.L. Vignoles (Eds.), *Handboook of identity theory and research* (pp. 149–175). Springer.

Chen, W.G., Schloesser, D., Arensdorf, A.M., Simmons, J.M., Cui, C., Valentino, R., Gnadt, J.W., Nielsen, L., St. Hillare-Clarke, C., Spruance, V., Horowitzz, T.S., Vallejo, Y.F., & Langecin, H.M. (2021). The emerging science of interoception: Sensing, integrating, interpreting, and regulating signals from within the self. *Trends Neurocience, 44*(1), 3–16. doi:10.1016/j.tins.2020.10.007

Cherry, K. (2022). What is brain plasticity? *Verywellmind*. https://www.verywellmind.com/what-is-brain-plasticity-2794886

Cherry, K. (2020). Introspection in psychology: Wundt's experimental technique. *Verywellmind*. https://www.verywellmind.com/what-is-introspection-2795252

Ciliberti, G. (2022, March 11). Purpose and the meaningful life – summary. *Philosophical Guidance*. https://philosophicalguidance.com/2022/03/11/purpose-and-the-meaingul-life-summary/

Cohen, P.R. & Levesque, H.J. (1990). Intention is choice with commitment. *Artificial Intelligence, 42*, 213–261. https://cs.stanford.edu/~epacuit/classes/lori-spr09/cohenlevesque-intention-aij90.pdf

Cotman, C.W. & Berchtold, N.C. (2002). Exercise: A behavioral intervention to enhance brain health and plasticity. *Trends in Neuroscience, 25*(6), 295–301.

Couch, S. (2015). What is intention? *Wild Gratitude*. https://www.wildgratitude.com/what-is-intention/

Crossman, A. (2018). Immersion definition: Cultural, language, and virtual. *ThoughtCo*. https://www.thoughtco.com/immersion-definition-3026534

Csikszentmihalyi, M. (1990). *Beyond boredom and anxiety: The experience of play in work and games*. Jossey-Bass.

Csikszentmihalyi, M. (1990). *Flow*. Harper.

Cushman, D.P. & Cahn, D.D. (1985). *Communication in interpersonal relationships*. SUNY Press.

Démuth, A. (2013). *Perception theories*. fftu.

Dictionary.com (2022a). Purpose. *Dictionary.com*. https://www.dictionary.com/browse/purpose

Dictionary.com (2022b). Pretence. *Dictionary.com*. https://www.dictionary.com/browse/pretence

Farlex (2022a). Boutons Terminaux. *The Free Dictionary, Medical*. https://medical-dictionary.thefreedictionary.com/boutons+terminaux

Farlex (2022b). Embody. *The Free Dictionary*. https://www.thefreedictionary.com/embody

Festinger, L. (1954). A theory of social comparison processes. *Human Relations*, 7(2), 117–132. https://www.humanscience.org/docs/Festinger%20(1954)%20A%20Theory%20of%20Social%20Comparison%20Processes.pdf

Fujimoto, A., Murray, E.A., & Rudebeck, P.H. (2021). Interaction between decision-making and interoceptive representations of bodily arousal in frontal cortex. *NIH*. https://www.ncbi.nlm.nih.gov/pmc/articles/PMC8536360/pdf/pnas.202014781.pdf

Harappa Diaries (2021, June 22). What is metacognition? *Harappa Diaries*. https://harappa.education/harappa-diaries/what-is-metacognition/

Harper, D. (2022). Introspection. *Online Etymology Dictionary*. https://www.etymonline.com/word/introspection

Held, R.M. & Durlach, N.I. (1992). Telepresence. *Presence: Teleoperators and Virtual Environments*, *1*(1), 102–112. https://www.deepdyve.com/lp/mit-press/telepresence-kNIrwUDqSm

Illis, L.S. (2012). Central nervous system regeneration does not occur. *Spinal Cord*, *50*, 259–263. https://www.nature.com/articles/sc2011132.pdf

Innocenti, G.M. (2022). Defining neuroplasticity. In M.J. Aminoff, F. Boller, & D.F. Swaab (Eds.), *Handbook of clinical neurology, 184* (pp. 3–18). Elsevier.

International Society for Presence Research (n.d.). Presence defined. *International Society for Presence Research*. https://ispr.info/about-presence-2/about-presence/

James, W. (1918). *The principles of psychology, vol. 1–2 (2 volumes in 1)*. Pantianos Classics.

Jung, C. (1971). *The portable Jung*. Penguin.

Kaduson, H.G. (2015). Play therapy across the lifespan: Infants, children, adolescents, and adults. In K.J. O'Connor, C.E. Schaefer, & L.D. Braverman (Eds.), *Handbook of play therapy*, 2nd ed. (pp. 327–341). Wiley.

Kenny, D.A. & West, T.V. (2008). Self-perception as interpersonal perception. In J.V. Wood, A. Tesser, & J.G. Holmes (Eds.), *The self and social relationships* (pp. 119–137). Taylor and Francis. 10.4324/9780203783061

Konorski, J. (1948). *Conditioned reflexes and neuron organization*. Cambridge University Press.

Kröger, S. & Watkins, B. (2021). Muscle spindle function in healthy and diseased muscle. *Skeletal Muscle*, *11*(3), 1–13. https://www.ncbi.nlm.nih.gov/pmc/articles/PMC7788844/pdf/13395_2020_Article_258.pdf

Kuhn, M.H. & McPartland, T.S. (1954). An empirical investigation of self-attitudes. *American Sociological Review*, *19*(1), 68–76. http://links.jstor.org/

sici?sici=0003-1224%28195402%2919%3A1%3C68%3AAEIOS%3E2.0.CO
%3B2-%23

Leitan, N.D. & Chaffey, L. (2014). Embodied cognition and its applications: A brief review. *Journal of Mind, Brain & Culture, 10*, 3–10. https://researchbank. swinburne.edu.au/items/e5f923e7-f9b7-4496-a4e0-f5d1365a4b4c/1/PDF %20%28Published%20version%29.pdf?.vi=save

Leslie, A. (1987). Pretence and representation: The origins of "theory of mind". *Psychological Review, 94*(4), 412–426.

Lieberman J.N. (1965). Playfulness and divergent thinking: An investigation of their relationship at the kindergarten level. *Journal of Genetic Psychology, 107*, 219–224.

Longo, M.R., Schüür, F., Kammers, M.P.M., Tsakiris, M., & Haggard, P. (2008). What is embodiment? A psychometric approach. *Cognition, 107*, 978–998.

Maslow, A. (1943). A theory of human motivation. *Psychological Review, 50*(4), 370–396.

Merriam-Webster (2022a). Intention. *Merriam-Webster.* https://www.merriam-webster.com/dictionary/intention

Merriam-Webster (2022b). Experience. *Merriam-Webster.* https://www.merriam-webster.com/dictionary/experience

Merriam-Webster (2022c). Immersion. *Merriam-Webster.* https://www.merriam-webster.com/dictionary/immersion

Merriam-Webster (2022d). Engross. *Merriam-Webster.* https://www.merriam-webster.com/dictionary/engross

Minsky, M. (1980). Telepresence. *Omni*, 45–51. https://web.media.mit.edu/~minsky/papers/Telepresence.html

Monti, A., Porciello, G., Panasiti, M.S., & Aglioti, S.M. (2021). The inside of me: Interoceptive constraints on the concept of self in neuroscience and clinical psychology. *Psychological Research.* https://link.springer.com/article/10.1007/s00426-021-01477-7

Moore, C. (2019). What is eudaimonia? Aristotle and eudaimonic well-being. *Postitive Psychology.* https://positivepsychology.com/eudaimonia/

NIH (2022). Brain basics: Know your brain. *National Institute of Neurological Disorders and Stroke.* https://www.ninds.nih.gov/health-information/patient-caregiver-education/brain-basics-know-your-brain

Nordquist, R. (2019, September 19). What is communication? The art of communicating and how to use it effectively. *ThoughtCo.* https://www.thoughtco.com/what-is-communication-1689877

Ossowska, K. (2021). Jerzy Konorski. *Polskie Towarzystwo Badań Ukladu Nerwowego.* https://ptbun.org.pl/en/jerzy-konorski-2/

Perera, A. (2020, September 4). Self-actualization. *SimplyPsychology.* https://www.simplypsychology.org/self-actualization.html

Perun, M. (2022). What is the importance of interpersonal relationships? *EscorpianAtl.* https://escorpionatl.com/what-is-importance-of-interpersonal-relationship

Piaget, J. (1962). *Play, dreams, and imitation in childhood.* Norton.

PressBooks (n.d.). What is cognition? *WSU.edu.* https://opentext.wsu.edu/psych105nusbaum/chapter/what-is-cognition/

Premack, D. & Woodruff, G. (1978). Does the chimpanzee have a theory of mind? *The Behavioral and Brain Sciences, 4,* 515–526.

Reference (2020, March 28). Why are communities important? *Reference.* https://www.reference.com/world-view/communities-important-7915d060a86ec7f3

Ritchie, D.G. (1892). What is reality? *The Philosophical Review, 1*(3), 265–283. https://www.jstor.org/stable/pdf/2175783.pdf

Rochat, P. (2003). Five levels of self-awareness as they unfold early in life. *Consciousness and Cognition, 12*(4), 717–731. 10.1016/s1053-8100(03)00081-3

Schaefer, C. & Greenberg, R. (1997). Measurement of playfulness: A neglected therapist variable. *International Journal of Play Therapy, 6*(2), 21–31.

Schalk, S. (2011). Self, other and other-self: going beyond the self/other binary in contemporary consciousness. *Journal of Comparative Research in Anthropology and Sociology, 2*(1), 197–210.

Shea, N. (2018). Metacognition and abstract concepts. *Royal Society Publishing.* https://royalsocietypublishing.org/journal/rstb

Sherrington, C.S. (1947). *Integrative action of the nervous system.* Cambridge.

Siegel, D.J. (2017). *Mind: A journey to the heart of being human.* Norton.

Siegel, D.J. (2012). *Pocket guide to interpersonal biology: An integrative handbook of the mind.* Norton.

Sluter, D. (2015). The importance of introspection: How often do you look in the mirror? *New England Construction.* https://www.neconstruction.com/blog/importance-of-introspection

Steuer, J. (1992). Defining virtual reality: Dimensions determining tele-presence. *Journal of Communication, 4*(2), 73–93.

Stahnisch, F.W. & Nitsch, R. (2002). Santiago Ramón y Cajal's concept of neuronal plasticity: The ambiguity lives on. *Trends in Neurosciences, 25*(11), 589–591.

Strigo, I.A. & Craig, A.D. (2016). Interoception, homeostatic emotions, and sympathovagal balance. *Philosophical Transactions B, 371.* https://www.ncbi.nlm.nih.gov/pmc/articles/PMC5062099/pdf/rstb20160010.pdf

Uttal, W.R. (1987). Mind, the psychobiology of. In G. Adelman (Ed.), *Encyclopedia of neuroscience, vol II* (pp. 672–674). Birkhäuser.

Varghese, N.K. (2018). *Existence and reality.* https://www.researchgate.net/publication/322682846

Vega, J.A. & Cobo, J. (2021, March 17). Structural and biological basis for proprioception. *IntechOpen.* https://pdfs.semanticscholar.org/5aee/7cfa83ec92f8d7f4fe7bd2590083a376c780.pdf?_ga=2.147202034.415650709.1663792239-1756145039.1657907263

Weisberg, D.S. (2015). Pretend play. *WIREs Cognitive Science, 6,* 249–261. doi: 10.1002/wcs.1341

4 Behavioral Neuroscience

The focus of this book is to discover and discuss the important concepts which contribute to the use of digital tools in mental health treatment. With a number of fundamental concepts fresh in our minds from Chapter 3, we continue on our journey by delving into information about portions of the brain, emotions, memory, and learning which have connections to our psychological foci.

Understanding what the brain's functions are and how the brain is internally connected to provide protection, integration, emotion, memory, cognition, metacognition, action, behavior, and so much more allows the clinician to proceed with evaluating digital tools for use in therapy and ultimately to understanding how these tools can be beneficial. This will not be a fully comprehensive list of the brain's components and functions, rather it is a list of the major structures and systems which contribute to cognitive and emotional functions of the brain. Similar to other conversations about technological advancements, knowledge of the brain has advanced tremendously in the past few decades. It is expected that some of this information will be replaced with new as we learn more.

As explored in Chapter 1, psychology has been "slow to change". One hypothesis for this approach is that professionals working in clinical psychology have a priority to "do no harm"; to guide and support their clients in ways that provide assistance and do not cause additional difficulties. That which is new has not been used for centuries and tried out by our discipline's forepeople; it has not passed through the rigor of disciplinary approvals over time. That which is new also brings forward questions of validity in ways approaches passed down by predecessors do not.

Certainly there are clinicians who have critically analyzed theories, approaches, and interventions in ways that have culminated into a solid foundation and repertoire that permeates all they do. However,

DOI: 10.4324/9781003171799-4

the majority of clinicians progressed through a graduate program as prescribed by the institution, met the requirements for their clinical hours, research, and licensure, and worked under a more seasoned clinician until independence was achieved. With the rigors of school, profession, and personal life moving into a face-paced, hectic phase of life, there is little space remaining for such deep analysis. It is understandable and expected.

What this often results in, however, is an acceptance of portions of the historical without the deeper understanding of the circumstances leading to its use or even dominance. As a fourth-grade student this author raised her hand and asked "why?" regarding a math concept. The teacher's response was to say, "it does not matter why, you just need to know how to do it". This dismissive, irresponsible approach sparked a lifetime of wanting to learn; to know why. As an adult, the question is still "why?", along with "how" and "what". These questions lead to professional deep dives into concepts, history, circumstance, politics, religion, and more, all with a focus on psychology and the "whys" of not only the field, but also the "whys" of humans.

In that spirit we have before us a chapter which has the intention of exploring the "whys" of the human brain, the impact of difficulties, how repair and assistance can be found/created/provided, and how digital tools can take part. It is important to take a biopsychosocial approach to humans and their ways of being and functioning, however, to be able to understand the sum of the parts, we must investigate the parts themselves. Neurology, with all the structures, networks, functions, and connections, is a foundation to function, emotion, and behavior. The mind is a window to the *self*, as well as the intertwining of *self* and other. The body is our vehicle to function, exploration, relationship, and communication. All have importance in psychology, therefore all must be considered and included.

Inclusion of the New

If we are going to include the new in our direct clinical work, caution is always important. The newest, most interesting hardware or software may initially engage, but it is the analysis and inclusion of the minutiae which allow us to confidently and competently incorporate the new and understand the why. An emphasis of knowing the "what, how, and why" regarding any approaches used in a clinical capacity allows the clinician the ability to move freely within well-understood professional boundaries and foundations. Knowing what the criteria and components are allows the clinician to vet the future new for clinical inclusion.

Brain, Mind, and Body

The connections of the brain, mind, and body are undeniable at this time in history. Remaining cognizant of the importance of these connections will allow the clinician to serve their clients well, as even if we think we are speaking to and with one portion of the brain, we are actually activating millions of neurons throughout the brain, mind, and body. Even if we are not aware of the magnitude of the process, holding space and recognition for the responses is important.

According to Damasio, the body provides the point of reference, the mind exists for an integrated internal system, and there has been an important interplay between the body and brain throughout evolution as a species and during an individual's development (2005). He states:

1 *The human brain and the rest of the body constitute an indissociable organism, integrated by means of mutually interactive biochemical and neural regulatory circuits (including endocrine, immune, and autonomic neural components);*
2 *The organism interacts with the environment as an ensemble: the interaction is neither of the body alone or of the brain alone;*
3 *The physiological operations that we call mind are derived from the structural and functional ensemble rather than from the brain alone: mental phenomena can be fully understood only in the context of an organism's interacting in an environment (2005, pp. xx–xxi).*

Brain and Mind

As discussed in Chapter 3, the distinction between the brain and the mind has been explored since the time of Hippocrates and Aristotle. Hippocrates believed the mind to be in the brain, and Aristotle believed it to be in the heart (Myers & DeWall, 2018). However, before we can contemplate the "where", we must investigate the "what". What is the mind, what is the brain, what is the body, and how do they come together to encompass the self? With a better understanding of each, we can begin to explore how each can be, and are, impacted, particularly when psychological assistance is needed. A holistic, full body approach can result in growth and change for the client, and competence and capability for the clinician.

The Mind

To expand the definition of the mind from Chapter 3, a neuroscience perspective considers the mind to be "as natural a function of brain circuit dynamics as digestion is of gastrointestinal actions, although the former is vastly more complex" (Panksepp, 1998, p. 59). Panksepp ponders that there is little scientific insight regarding the fundamental sources of mind and behavior that words can provide, rather, advances in neuroanatomy, neurophysiology, and neurochemistry can all contribute to our understandings moving forward (1998). Neuroscience wants to understand the structures, their relationships, their functions, and their communications in order to further understand human emotion and behavior.

Brain

The brain is a complex and vital organ within the human body. While we still have much to learn, great advancements have been made toward understanding the structures, components, networks, and pathways of the brain. We speak of the brain as a static organ, one which is stable and predictable, however, it is often not. Neural firing patterns fluctuate from at least 4–100 times per second, and axons connect throughout the body in somewhat unpredictable ways thus providing a plethora of possible actions and reactions (Badenoch, 2008). Just as clinicians say "if you've met one person with x (a diagnosis), then you've met one person with x", we would have to speak in terms of a constellation of specifics from any given moment to speak precisely about the brain's function. Therefore, by default we are speaking of a complex and varying dynamic in a more concrete and static way, yet understanding that this is a necessary reality for understanding the complexities.

Adult human brains have been found to have 86.1±8.1 billion NeuN-positive cells (known as neurons) as of 2009 (Azevedo et al., 2009). The year is given for reference, as 100 billion was previously believed and Azevedo et al.'s research showed otherwise. Future research may yield a different number over time. One may wonder why it matters. The response is that it matters a great deal because we assign a variety of attributes to humans based on previous assumptions and beliefs. Many theories are based on the concept that a larger brain in humans (comparative to body size) is attributed to intellectual superiority. A belief in superiority separates us from other primates (and other animals) and reduces the generalizability of research findings, along with the further understanding of the brain.

> *With only 19% of all neurons located in the cerebral cortex, greater cortical size (representing 82% of total brain mass) in humans compared with other primates does not reflect an increased relative number of cortical neurons. The ratios between glial cells and neurons in the human brain structures are similar to those found in other primates, and their numbers of cells match those expected for a primate of human proportions. These findings challenge the common view that humans stand out from other primates in their brain composition and indicate that, with regard to numbers of neuronal and nonneuronal cells, the human brain is an isometrically scaled-up primate brain.*
>
> (Azevedo et al., 2009, p. 535)

Additionally, it matters because it exemplifies that although information can change throughout time, humans tend to hold on to historical information and potentially continue to misassign meaning – as we have discussed earlier in this text.

Clinical Relevance

When working with a client, a mental health clinician is utilizing their theoretical framework and experience to conceptualize the client, their past experiences, present experiences, world view (how they see the world and themselves in it), relationship skills, styles, and approaches, interaction skills, styles, and approaches, strategic skills, needs, desires, hopes, goals, and so much more. How does the client define many of the concepts from Chapter 3 for themselves? For instance, how do they experience and interpret their own self, experience of interoception, identification, representation, reality, and more. How can we conceptualize both how they understand themselves and how we understand them in a way that assists them with the therapeutic goals? Once conceptualized, even as hypotheses, how do we utilize interventions to learn more and impact their emotions, memory, and learning in therapeutically productive ways? What are the mechanisms involved and how do we access them; how do we best assist our clients? What are the paths to accessing, processing, and organizing that which is necessary for the client to move forward?

Continuing to learn about the self, brain, mind, and body are imperative to continuing to understand the ways we can access and assist our clients with their psychological difficulties. Asking the client to look inward, as clinicians should do as well, informs the identification, representation, and theory of mind for us all.

On Being Human

The brain and the body include intricate systems within. There are currently 7.9 billion people in the world (Worldometer, 2022). It is amazing how billions of humans can have such variety and such consistency at the same time. Our physical features can vary greatly, yet the inner workings of the body are predominately the same. Even structures in the brain can vary in size, shape, and appearance, yet have very similar function (assuming health). If we sit with that for a moment, it is truly astonishing and phenomenal.

As mental health professionals, we are tasked with understanding the intricacies of another human. Experiences, history, and perspectives may create an innumerable number of complexities within the emotional and behavioral presentations and concerns, but the processes by which we access them can be narrowed down quite effectively. Informed by education, experience, and a theoretical base, clinicians can identify interventions which elicit responses that contribute to the psychological growth of the client.

Beyond the verbal and non-verbal information our clients provide, mental health clinicians who are knowledgeable regarding the brain structure and functions will provide a holistic conceptualization of the difficulties the client is experiencing. Our "do no harm" also includes being as knowledgeable, inquisitive, and exploratory as is necessary to properly conceptualize and provide services to those who seek them.

To understand the relative commonalities of being human, we will define and review the brain structures involved in this clinical pursuit. If we understand the ways in which the brain and body conceptualize, process, communicate, and react, then we can expertly identify clinical agents of change and employ interventions which move the client toward psychological health.

Brain and Body

A few component definitions:

- Gray matter – nerve or neural cell bodies of the brain
- White matter – composed of nerve fibers, or axons, coated in myelin, which connect nerve cells within the brain (Heerema, 2021).

- Glia – cells which support and protect neurons in the gray matter, these are cells and not neurons; there are a variety of types including astrocytes, oligondendrocytes, and microglia. Astrocytes are believed to be key components of synapses and impact information processing (Queensland Brain Institute, 2017).
- Axons – interconnections in the white matter, protected by the glial cells; they will redirect their growth toward their normal targets, even when displaced (Jackson, 1987). A specialize portion of the neuron which transmits information form the soma and dendrites to the presynaptic terminals (Waxman, 1987).
- Gyri (Gyrus) – the convolutions or ridges of the cerebral cortex surface which are named according to their location (Difference Between, 2014).
- Sulci (Sulcus) – grooves or fissures on the cortex surface of the brain, found between the gyri and named according to their location (Difference Between, 2014).
- Myelin – an electric insulator made of protein and fatty substances which speeds up the signals between cells and creates the white color of white matter (Medline Plus, n.d.)
- Neuron – a nerve cell with three definable parts: cell body (soma, including a nucleus and cytoplasm), dendrites, and axons. Most neurons have one axon and multiple dendrites. They do not undergo mitosis, and therefore do not regenerate except in the granule cells of the cerebellar cortex and dentata fascia in the hippocampal formation (Palay & Chan-Palay, 1987).

Nervous Systems

There are two primary nervous systems within the human body: the central (CNS) and the peripheral (PNS). The central nervous system includes the brain and spinal cord. The CNS is considered the command center of the human body. The PNS is an intricate system of nerves which connect the rest of the body to the CNS. The PNS can be divided into the somatic and autonomic systems. Somatic functions are those commanded by the body in an intentional way, i.e., to move a certain way or hold one's breath. Autonomic functions are involuntary, i.e., breathing and pumping blood throughout the body (Siegel, 2012).

These essential systems gather information from both inside and outside the body so the pertinent response can be dispatched. The informational messages travel through the body via neuronal networks; electronic impulses traveling from neuron to neuron, through the soma (cell body), axon, and dendrites, to their final destination. The communication path is one directional. Sensory neurons transmit information from the body to the brain and motor neurons transmit from the brain to the body (Stevens, 2022).

The direction of the information being communicated: from inside the body or from outside the body; from the body to the brain or the brain to the body, informs us about the stimuli that the client is attending to and receiving information from. We will certainly not be able to determine the nervous system components within a session, but it is important to conceptualize the possible origins of information, where and how it travels, and what the impact might be on the client.

Additionally, the autonomic and somatic nervous systems have important functions. Along with the amygdala, prefrontal cortex, and the hypothalamus, the autonomic nervous system (ANS) has a large role in regulation (Badenoch, 2008). When the body's homeostasis is compromised, and therefore dysregulated, the ANS determines whether or not the body needs to increase or decrease its response systems to regain homeostasis. The Window of Tolerance, described by Siegel, is achieved when there is balance between the sympathetic and parasympathetic nervous systems (1999).

The ANS is a part of the peripheral nervous system and regulates processes within the body without conscious intention. This system maintains bidirectional communication between the brainstem and organs such as the heart, liver, and intestines (Siegel, 2012). ANS dysregulation and dysfunction can be caused by chronic stress and impact the digestive, neuroendocrine, cardiovascular, and respiratory systems, as well as contribute to psychiatric disorders (Daniela et al., 2022).

The ANS is divided further into three additional branches: the sympathetic, parasympathetic, and enteric nervous systems (Cherry, 2021a). The sympathetic and parasympathetic systems are frequently referred to in psychological environments, particularly in terms of emotional regulation. When these systems are not working well together it can result in an autonomic disorder called dysautonomia (Cherry, 2021a).

Siegel (2012) and Badenoch (2008) both liken the sympathetic system to the accelerator of a car and the parasympathetic to the brakes of a car. The sympathetic system arouses and excites; respiration, heart rate, states of alertness, and sweating can all increase due to the arousal of this system. Activation of the sympathetic system generates the resources for the fight-flight-freeze response to perceived threat (Siegel, 2012). The sympathetic system quickly responds and mobilizes the body for action (Cherry, 2021a). Norepinephrine, epinephrine, and dopamine are the primary neurotransmitters in the sympathetic system.

Norepinephrine is released by postganglionic neurons and this process activates the receptors on a target organ and signals the need to "jump" into action. This is important in psychology because norepinephrine impacts mood, arousal, memory, learning, metabolism, and blood flow. Additionally, dopamine is involved in memory, behavior, cognition, pleasure, personality, movement, and sleep. A deficiency in these sympathetic neurotransmitters can influence depression, anxiety, bipolar, and addiction disorders and an excess is related to schizophrenia (Daniela et al., 2022).

The parasympathetic system inhibits; respiration, heart rate, states of alertness, and sweating can all decrease due to this system (Siegel, 2012). This inhibition serves to conserve resources and maintain normal bodily functions. (Cherry, 2021a). The primary neurotransmitter of the parasympathetic system is acetylcholine (Ach), which participates in the regulation of learning, memory, cognition, arousal, and moderating sensory information (Daniela et al., 2022).

The somatic nervous system (SNS) is vital in the initiation and control of voluntary movements of the body. This is a central system used in proprioception. The SNS is also involved in processing external sensory stimuli, such as hearing, touch, smell, and sight (Cherry, 2021b). There are two primary types of neurons in the SNS: sensory or afferent neurons and motor or efferent neurons.

Sensory neurons carry information from the body to the central nervous system. Through a process called sensory transduction, the sensory neurons convert a sensory stimulus into an electrical message and communicated by the neurons (Oxford Scholarship, 2022). Motor neurons are the largest neurons in the central nervous system. These neurons activate muscle fibers and cause them to contract. Located within the brainstem and spinal cord, they impact upward toward the brain and the lower spinal roots (Burke, 1987).

The enteric nervous system is located in the gastrointestinal tract which extends from the esophagus to the rectum. This system of sensory, motor, and interneurons and regulates digestive functions. Sometimes referred to as the "second brain" and responds to digested food and drink by processing the intake or rejecting it due to bacteria or other issues (Tresca, 2021). This is the mechanism by which we refer to the brain-gut connection.

The nervous systems impact critical responses in the body, whether it be transporting information to or from the brain. The information that is communicated, processed, and then acted upon within this complex system impacts our safety, arousal, memory, learning, cognition, pleasure, movement, and behavior.

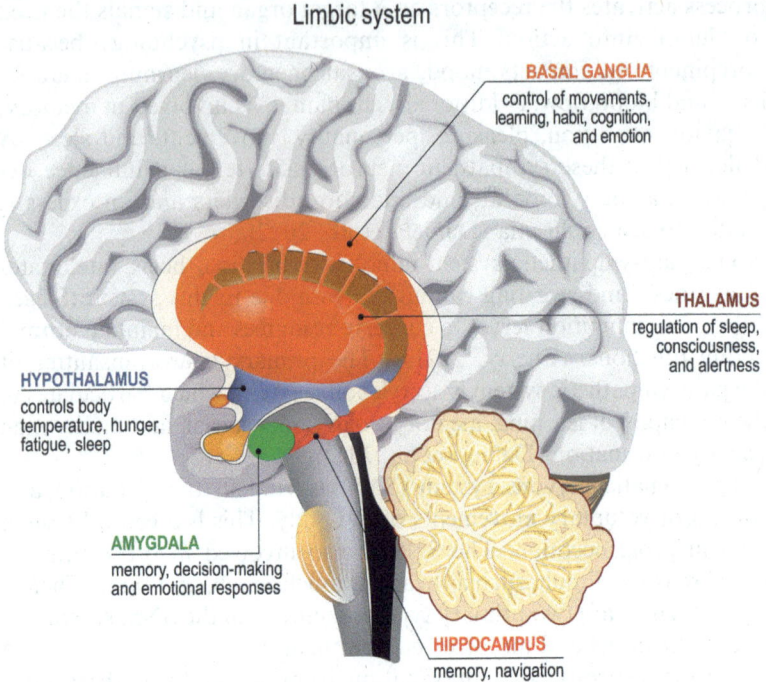

Cerebral Cortex and Lobes of the Brain

We can begin with an overview of MacLean's triunal approach to the brain, albeit a simplified approach. MacLean identified three evolutionary layers of the brain: neomammalian (neocortex), old mammalian (limbic), and reptilian (basal ganglia) (MacLean, 1970, 1985). With each layer believed to reflect long periods of stability in brain evolution, the triune approach is an relatively simplistic beginning to our journey.

Within the triune approach, the neomammalian or neocortex is believed to generate logical thought, higher cognitive functioning, and reasoning. The old mammalian brain includes the limbic system. The limbic system is believed to add behavioral and psychological elements, including social emotions, bonding, playfulness, nurturance, and separation distress. The reptilian portion or basal ganglia of the brain is the core of the brain and includes the most primitive emotional processes such as sexuality, dominance, eating, and exploring (Panskepp, 1998).

The brain is believed to have areas of higher cortical and cognitive functioning, and those which are more primitive. However, the areas are interconnected and we continue to learn more about the functions and relationship of all the areas.

The Cerebral Cortex

The cerebral cortex is the outer most layer of the brain that is unique to human beings. It is also known as the neocortex and the neo-mammalian cortex (Siegel, 2012). It consists of gray matter and is only a few millimeters or about 6 cells thick which is filled with columns of "highly linked neuronal clusters" (Siegel, 2012, p. AI-20). Functions such as information processing, language, consciousness, imagination, higher-order thinking, memory, perception, reasoning, relationship, and sensation are associated with the cerebral cortex (Cherry, 2021c; Badenoch, 2008).

The most rostral, or furthest foreword, portion of the cerebral cortex is the prefrontal cortex. It appears that this cortex is involved in organizing goal-directed behavior as well as information processing functions such as thinking, reasoning, and perceiving (Siegel, 2012). The prefrontal cortex communicates reciprocally (both directions) with the anterior and dorsal nuclei of the thalamus and several sensory processing areas (somatic, auditory, olfactory, and visual) of the posterior association cortex, with limbic areas such as the hypothalamus, amygdala, and the hippocampus (memory, emotion, and motivation), and the motor areas (basal ganglia, thalamus, and cerebellum). (Fuster, 1987). The details of this matter because of the functions of the hypothalamus, amygdala, and hippocampus which will be discussed later in the chapter.

The cerebral cortex has been divided into four lobes: frontal, parietal, temporal, and occipital. The four lobes are then divided into three areas of functioning: sensory, motor, and association (Washmuth, 2022). We are working through the structures of the brain to identify the areas where key psychologically engaged functions are involved.

Lobes of the Cerebral Cortex and Areas of Functioning

Occipital lobe – The occipital lobe is in the back of the brain and integrates portions of visual information (such as color, spatial orientation, motion of an object, face recognition, depth perception, and environment mapping) into whole images (Badenoch, 2008;

Washmuth, 2022). The primary visual cortex is located in this lobe and therefore processes and interprets visual information and stimuli from the retinas of the eyes. Processing visual information includes determining what something is through the ventral stream pathway and where something is through the ventral stream pathway. The dorsal stream will send the information to the parietal lobe and ventral to the temporal lobe. This process assists with determining if something is a friend or foe (Stevens, 2022). Damage to the occipital lobe is associated with difficulties recognizing words, colors, and objects (Cherry, 2021c).

Parietal lobe – The parietal lobe processes sensory information through the somatosensory cortex, such as temperature, pain, pressure, and touch and is located in the midbrain section (Badenoch, 2008; Cherry, 2021c). Additionally, this lobe processes components of understanding speech and reading (Badenoch, 2008). The precuneus is located in the parietal lobe and is involved in proprioception as well as visuospatial perception (Stevens, 2022). Damage to this lobe can cause issues with sensory perception, vision issues, left-side neglect, spatial relations and body image (Badenoch, 2008; Flint Rehab, 2020).

Temporal Parietal Junction – The temporal and parietal lobes meet at the temporal parietal junction (TPJ). Language, memory, attention, social cognition, and theory of mind have been associated with the TPJ (Van Overwalle, 2009; Stevens, 2022).

Temporal lobe – The temporal lobe is home to a number of important brain structures. The primary auditory cortex is located in the temporal lobe and necessary to interpret parts of language and sounds. Additional roles include emotions, memory, smell, and hearing (Washmuth, 2022). The hippocampus is also located here and associated with the formation of memories. Neural components associated with fear, rage and lust, possibly due to the connection of this lobe to regions of the amygdala (Panskepp, 1998). Damage to this lobe can lead to memory, speech perception, and language skill difficulties (Cherry, 2021c).

Frontal lobe – Located in the front portion of the brain, the frontal lobe is associated with expressive language, motor skills, reasoning, concentration, judgment, creativity, personality, abstract thinking, emotional regulation, social skills, and a higher-level cognition and planning (Badenoch, 2008; Siegel, 2012; Washmuth, 2022). It is sometimes referred to as the associational cortex due to the "linkages among widely interconnected processes fundamental to higher thinking and planning" (Siegel, 2012, p AI-34). Damage to this portion of the brain can result in difficulties with risk taking, attention, socialization, and sexual habits. The motor cortex lies at the rear portion of the frontal lobe (Cherry, 2021c).

The three areas of functioning are dispersed throughout the cerebral cortex and not relegated to one area. The sensory area processes hearing, smell, pain, and touch. The motor area "initiates and controls movements of the body such as walking or moving the arms and hands while eating" (Washmuth, 2022, para 4). The association area includes involvement with functions such as language, decision-making, planning, and cognition (Washmuth, 2022).

Although the brain has been defined in terms of regions, it is a highly interconnected organ whose impact reaches throughout via magical dendritic connections. Conceptualizing the brain in more of a systems perspective than individualistic is important for psychological work.

Lower to Higher Brain Regions

Brainstem – Located in the base of the brain, the brainstem includes clusters of neurons which activate the fight-flight-freeze reflexes and regulate the cardiac, respiratory, and central nervous systems (Sciacca et al., 2019). The medulla oblongata, pons, and midbrain are included in the brainstem. This area regulates body temperature, heart rate, and breathing (Siegel, 2012).

Midbrain – At the top of the brainstem is the midbrain. Small, but mighty, the midbrain is believed to be a relay station for auditory and visual information, and the controls for eye movement (Cherry, 2021c). The neurotransmitter dopamine is produced in the substantia nigra of the midbrain to be distributed throughout the brain (Stevens, 2022; Cherry, 2021c). As mentioned earlier, dopamine is involved with memory, behavior, cognition, pleasure, personality, movement, and sleep.

Medulla Oblongata – The medulla oblongata, or medulla, is located beneath the pons, above the spinal cord and in the lower part of the brainstem. The medulla controls autonomic functions such as blood pressure, heart rate, and breathing (Cherry, 2021c).

Pons – The pons is considered part of the upper brainstem. Connecting the cerebellum to the rest of the brain, the pons is involved in basic functions such as breathing and sleeping (Stevens, 2022). Interestingly, the pons includes the raphe nuclei (serotonin), ventral tegmental area (dopamine), and locus coeruleus (norepinephrine) which are involved in mood and emotion (Venkatraman et al., 2017;

Stevens, 2022). Venkatraman et al. state: "the human brainstem contributes to the evaluation of sensory information and triggers fixed-action pattern responses that together constitute the finely differentiated spectrum of possible emotions" (2017, p. 1).

Cerebellum – The cerebellum is located behind the top of the brainstem at the bottom of the brain. It is sometimes referred to as the "little brain" due to its shape and small lobes. This small but important area of the brain coordinates movement, walking, and balance via information relayed from sensory neurons, auditory and visual systems, and the inner ear (Cherry, 2021c). Motor learning is also associated with the cerebellum, such as memorization of the process to drive a car, type on a keyboard without looking, and more. Damage to the cerebellum has been found to impact speech, language, executive function, visuospatial cognition, and changes in emotion and has been named cerebellar cognitive affective syndrome, or Schmahmann's syndrome (Schmahmann et al., 2019).

Insular Cortex – The insular cortex, or insula, is housed inside the Sylvain fissure, which separates the frontal, temporal, and parietal lobes; it is nestled in the center of many important structures. The insula's purpose is critical to understanding one's own self and emotions; without it one would not be able to differentiate between emotions which complicates cognition, decision-making, planning, reacting, etc. (Human Mind, 2022). The insula can be thought of as the center of self-awareness, interoception, and Theory of Mind (Siegel, 2012). Critical to social relationships, the VENs neurons in the insula are responsible for our ability to read social cues. Damage to the insula, commonly in conjunction with damage to the limbic system, can contribute to mental illness and compulsivity (Human Mind, 2022).

The insula is dependent upon the limbic system to connect and relay signals; it connects higher cortical areas with bodily processes (Human Mind, 2022). The information from the body travels up the spinal cord, and vagal nerve, to the brainstem and then the insula (Siegel, 2012). Per Badenoch, "Researchers believe that the streams of information converging here provide an emotionally relevant context for sensory information" (2008, p. 17).

Once believed to be focused purely on the functions of the body, modern technologies have allowed us to understand more about the interconnectedness and multi-function purpose of the lower brain regions, particularly in terms of self, Theory of Mind, interoception, speech, language, emotion, pleasure, proprioception, and cognition.

ANATOMY OF THE BRAIN

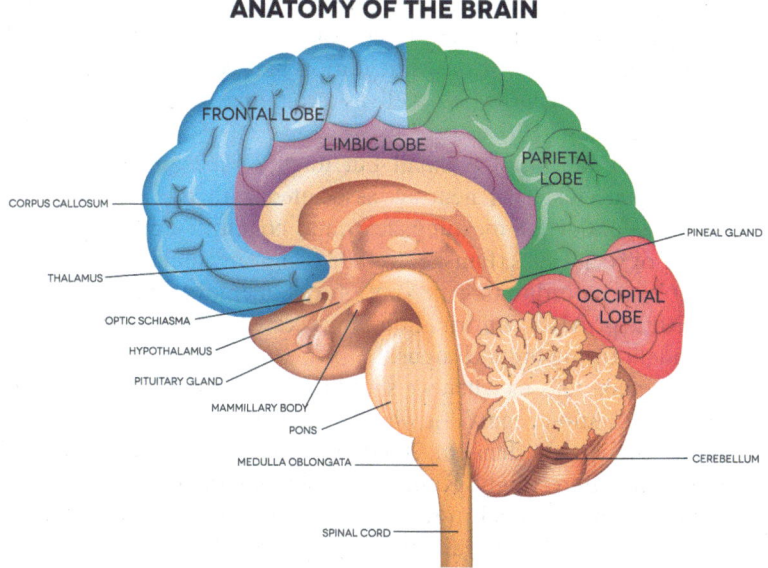

Limbic System

The limbic system contributes to memory, motivation, and learning, as well as response, regulation, attachment, behavior, and attention. Certainly all the components of the brain we have discussed thus far are critical, and, the limbic system includes structures which have received center-stage status in behavioral neurobiology.

Located in the medial temporal lobe, the center of the brain, the limbic system includes the amygdala and hippocampus, a duo which coordinates between the body, and the higher and lower portions of the brain. Thought to be essential for attachment, this area integrates processes such as social signals, emotional activation, and the appraisal of meaning (Siegel, 2012).

Hypothalamus – Near the pituitary at the base of the brain, this grouping of nuclei is another connector with many other regions. The hypothalamus is responsible for the regulation of body temperature regulation, circadian rhythms, hunger, thirst, emotions, and hormones (Cherry, 2021c; Siegel, 2012). By controlling the secretion of hormones, the hypothalamus maintains control over many bodily functions (Cherry, 2021c).

Amygdala – The amygdala is located in the rostromedial part of the temporal lobe and connects to the corpus striatum. It is sometimes thought of as part of the basal ganglia, although it is distinct. Believed to be involved in the "integration and control of emotional and autonomic behaviors" as well as "cognitive functions such as memory processing" (Price, 1987, p. 41).

This part of the brain is small but mighty. The amygdala is an almond-shaped cluster of neurons associated with the activation of emotion, evaluation of meaning, learning, cognitive appraisals, and processing of social cues (Panskepp, 1998). The amygdala also "plays a crucial role in coordinating perceptions of memory and behavior" (Siegel, 2012, p. AI-4). Information is processed and then relayed by the amygdala to the hippocampus.

The amygdala tells us when we should pay attention and makes an initial determination regarding whether or not situations are safe or not, good or bad (Badenoch, 2008). We can then respond to perceived threat. Interestingly, Rafal et al., demonstrated that there is a subcortical pathway which transmits information when the pulvinar activates (nucleus of the thalamus) to the amygdala that is not dependent upon the primary visual cortex (2014), which means threatening visual stimuli was not processed by the visual cortex. It is possible that due to the type of stimuli (threatening) the body bypassed the highe-order processing in favor of needing a determination, therefore this pathway to the amygdala was activated. This may have deep implications within psychology as it may mean that a stimulus that is determined to be a threat could be reacted to without higher-order thinking directly involved. In psychology, it may behoove us to expose clients to a predefined level of perceived threat so we can pause mid process to encourage and guide toward the higher-order processing of the situation.

Thalamus – The thalamus is situated on the top of the brainstem and serves as a relay station which passes emotional, sensory, attentional, and movement information to the cerebral cortex (Arend et al., 2015; Siegel, 2012; Cherry, 2021c). This communication is bidirectional, with the cerebral cortex also passing along information to the thalamus to be sent to other systems within the body (Cherry, 2021c). The thalamus can be likened to the hub of a transit station, with messages coming and going to multiple destinations.

The pulvinar nucleus is the largest in the thalamus and is believed to be strongly connected with the visual cortex (Arend et al., 2014). Modulating emotion and attention processes through the colliculo-pulvino-amygdalar pathway, the pulvinar has an important role in "coordinating multimodal signals and highlighting information that is significant to the individual" (Arend et al., 2014, p. 191; Padmala et al., 2010). The pulvinar is involved in working memory and binds "visual objects to their respective emotional value during working memory updating" (Arend et al., 2014, p. 195; Grecucci et al., 2010). Following in Rafal et al.'s work with the amygdala, the thalamus has been found to coactivate with visual areas, but only in a minimal way as the pulvinar can act independently as well (Barron et al., 2015).

Hippocampus – The hippocampus is predominately associated with encoding and recalling memories and emotional responses (Cherry, 2021c). It is shaped like a seahorse and resides in the limbic area of the medial temporal lobe (Siegel, 2012). The hippocampus has a central role "in flexible forms of memory, in the recall of facts and auto-biographical details. It gives the brain a sense of self in space and in time, regulates the order of perceptual categorizations, and links mental representations to emotional appraisal centers" (Siegel, 2012, p. AI-36).

Some critical information we now know about the memory encoding and recalling of the hippocampus includes what we remember and how we remember it. Historically it was believed that memory retrieval was similar to pulling a book of a library shelf; it was preserved in a relatively stable state when it was stored. However, new (and exciting) findings indicate otherwise (Stevens, 2022). Memory recall has been questioned for years, as shown in the difficulty people have recalling crime scene events, etc. Humans also have a tendency to remember positive events more than negative, and when we recall the negative, we tend to forget how bad they really were (for example, if we remembered the reality of a difficult situation, far fewer humans would ever be born).

Barry & Maguire demonstrated that the hippocampus does not recall the memory, rather it reconstructs it (2019). The prefrontal cortex and the hippocampus work together, bidirectionally, and jointly reconstruct a memory for "recall" (Eichenbaum, 2017; Stevens, 2022).

When recalling a memory, the brain uses heuristics in constructing that event. If you're trying to remember going to grandma's house for Thanksgiving five years ago, the brain appears to recreate that picture from all of the times at grandma's house, making it difficult to remember if that new painting came last year or has been there for ten years.

(Stevens, 2022, p. 39.)

This has far reaching implications for mental health treatment. A concept Stevens calls "affect reconsolidation" will be discussed later in this text. Perceptions of experiences are what we carry, what impacts us over time, and what we integrate into our sense of self, our interoception, and Theory of Mind.

The hypothalamus, amygdala, thalamus, and hippocampus serve many purposes within the human brain: memory, motivation, and learning, response, regulation, attachment, behavior, and attention. Continuing to explore not only the structural components of the brain through improving technologies, but also expanding our understanding of the human experience and process while applying the learning to psychological concepts and approaches will improve the care we provide.

Tectum – The tectum contains the corpora quadrigemina, which in turn contains two colliculi nerve clusters, the superior and the inferior (Doherty, 2021). The superior colliculus (SC) and the inferior colliculus (IC) are located in the rear portion of the midbrain. Both of these structures will be discussed with clinical implications later in the text.

Superior Colliculus – Visual signals are processed through the superior colliculus prior to being channeled to the occipital lobe. Eye movements are also controlled by the SC.

Inferior Colliculus – Auditory signals are processed through the inferior colliculus prior to being channeled through the thalamus, then to the auditory cortex in the temporal lobe. Additionally, the IC is responsible for discriminating pitch and rhythm, orienting the body toward stimuli, and the startle response (Doherty, 2021).

The superior and inferior colliculi process visual and auditory signals prior to being transmitted to other portions of the brain; what we attend to, what we preliminarily perceive as scary and/or threatening, is decided on, in part, by these structures. These decisions impact our actions and reactions, and depending on the perceived level of danger, may or may not initially involve the frontal lobe.

Networks

There are a number of identified networks in the brain. Here we will discuss two of the most applicable networks for our purpose: the default mode network and the task positive network.

Default Mode Network (DMN) (task-negative network) –

The DMN became a larger focus in the 21st century after it was discovered that a particular portion of the brain had reduced activation during executive function task-related activities (Greicius et al.,

2003; Mohan et al., 2016; Buckner et al., 2008; Raichle, 2015). Historically, this name denotes the "resting brain"; the activity of the brain when it is not actively working on something else, hence "default". Originally this was believed to be a time when the brain was less active and using minimal energy. However, with low-frequency oscillations of around one fluctuation per second, the DMN is actually most active when the rest of the brain is at rest (Pressman, 2018). The DMN is a network within the intrinsic connectivity networks (ICNs), and is the most well-known of the ICNs.

The DMN is a highly active network which includes the medial temporal lobe, the medial prefrontal cortex, the posterior cingulate cortex, ventral precuneus, and portions of the parietal cortex. Believed to a network which is comprised of a collection of smaller networks, the DMN appears to be associated with different aspects of memory, theory of mind, and internal thought integration (Pressman, 2018).

The DMN is particularly specialized for "self-referential thinking" (Stevens, 2022, p. 43). When we are not actively working on or toward something else, the mind tends to think about the self; what did I do, need to do, think feel, remember, desire, etc. William James referred to this as a "stream of consciousness" (1918). So while the initial thought was that the mind was in a resting state, in reality, the mind is active with introspection, interospection, theory of mind, remembering the past, and planning for the future when the default mode network is active (Chan & Siegel, 2018; Hull, 2021) MRI imaging of a person who is experiencing a depressive state shows that the DMN is very active, presumably the person is thinking, ruminating, etc. Conversely, activities such as mindful meditation can relax the DMN (Stevens, 2022)

Central Executive Network (CEN) (task positive network) – The central executive network becomes active when the brain is focused on a task, performance, and/or action. When the CEN is active, the DMN shows a decrease in activation (Greicius et al., 2003). Involved in "demanding cognitive tasks, like complex problem solving, working memory, and executive functioning tasks", the CEN has a large functional connectivity with other portions of the brain (Stevens, 2022, p. 43). The CEN appears to be a flexible hub which acts as a problem-solver and connects with different neural networks depending on the complex task needs (Zanto & Gazzaley, 2013; Stevens, 2022).

Everything in life moves us toward homeostasis; too much time with an active DMN can result in anxiety, depression, wallow; too much time with the CEN active and one can lack self-knowledge, insight, and most likely difficulty in relationships. As clinicians who are aware of these network shifts, we can work with our clients toward homeostasis; toward balance. When we explore whether or not their DMN or CEN might be "in charge" or activated, we can respond with appropriate guidance and interventions. We might give a person with an activated DMN an intentional task, bring them out of their internal state. A person with an active CEN may need to find ways to move more inward; to self-reflect and focus on the moment.

The default mode network and central executive network work beautifully in tandem to move our brain, mind, and body toward balance and homeostasis. Incorporating this into our therapeutic work helps us and our clients to understand what is needed to move toward the center.

Armed with the knowledge of the brain, mind, and body, the clinician can answer many more of the "whys and hows" within psychology. This information can be applied to all that we do, and all that will come in the future so that the new does not need to be feared, rather, it can be evaluated utilizing the knowledge of need and processes of change within humans. This is a base that will continue to grow as we learn more. This is a base that allows us to have comfort and competence in the "what"; in the interventions and interactions within the therapeutic process. Applying these concepts to the vetting and inclusion of digital tools within clinical psychology broadens our base and opens our discipline to the expansive power of what is before us.

References

Arend, I., Henik, A., & Okon-Singer (2015). Dissociating emotion and attention functions in the pulvinar nucleus of the thalamus. *American Psychological Association, 29*(2), 191–196.

Azevedo, F.A.C., Carvalho, L.R.B., Grinberg, L.T., Farfel, J.M., Ferretti, R.E.L., Leite, R.E.P., Filho, W.J., Lent, R., & Herculano-Houzel, S. (2009). Equal numbers of neuronal and nonneuronal cells make the human brain an isometrically scaled-up primate brain. *The Journal of Comparative Neurology, 513*, 532–541.

Badenoch, B. (2008). *Being a brain-wise therapist: A practical guide to interpersonal biology.* Norton.

Barron, D.S., Eickhoff, S.B., Cos, M., & Fox, P.T. (2015). Human pulvinar functional organization and connectivity. *Human Brain Mapping, 36*, 2417–2431. https://onlinelibrary.wiley.com/doi/epdf/10.1002/hbm.22781

Barry, D.N., & Maguire, E.A. (2019). Remote memory and the hippocampus: A constructive critique. *Trends in Cognitive Sciences, 23*(2), 128–142.

Buckner, R.L., Andrews-Hanna, J.R., & Schacter, D.L. (2008). The brain's default network: Anatomy, function, and relevance to disease. *New York Academy of Sciences, 1124*, 1–38.

Burke, R.E. (1987). Motoneurons. In G. Adelman (Ed.), *Encyclopedia of neuroscience, vol II* (pp. 688–690). Birkhäuser.

Chan, A., & Siegel, D. (2018). Play and the default mode network: Interpersonal neurobiology, self, and creativity. In T. Marks-Tarlow, M. Solomon, & D.J. Siegel (Eds.), *Play and creativity in psychotherapy* (pp. 39–63). W.W. Norton.

Cherry, K. (2021a, April 17). What is the autonomic nervous system? *Verywellmind.* https://www.verywellmind.com/what-is-the-autonomic-nervous-system-2794823

Cherry, K. (2021b, April 14). What is the somatic nervous system? *Verywellmind.* https://www.verywellmind.com/what-is-the-somatic-nervous-system-2795866

Cherry, K. (2021c, June 8). Parts of the brain. *Verywellmind.* https://www.verywellmind.com/the-anatomy-of-the-brain-2794895

Damasio, A. (2005). *Descartes' error: Emotion, reason, and the human brain.* Penguin.

Daniela, M., Catalina, L., Ille, O., Paula, M., Daniel-Andrei, O., & Ioana, B. (2022). Effects of exercise training on the autonomic nervous system with a focus on anti-inflammatory and antioxidants effects. *Antioxidants, 11*(350), 1–34.

Difference Between (2014, October 23). Difference between gyri and sulci. *Difference Between.* https://www.differencebetween.com/difference-between-gyri-and-vs-sulci

Doherty, C. (2021, February 10). The anatomy of the midbrain: Also called the mesencephalon. *Verywellhealth.* https://www.verywellhealth.com/midbrain-anatomy-5093684

Eckman, P. (2003). *Emotions revealed: Recognizing faces and feelings to improve communication and emotional life.* Times.

Eichenbaum, J. (2017). Prefrontal-hippocampal interactions in episodic memory. *Nature Reviews Neuroscience, 18*(9), 547–558.

Flint Rehab (2020, May 21). Parietal lobe damage: Understanding symptoms and treatments. *Flint Rehab.* https://www.flintrehab.com/parietal-lobe-damage/

Fuster, J.M. (1987). Prefrontal cortex. In G. Adelman (Ed.), *Encyclopedia of neuroscience, vol II* (pp. 972–975). Birkhäuser.

Grecucci, A., Soto, D., Rumiati, R.I., Humphreys, G.W., & Rotshtein, P. (2010). The inter-correlations between verbal working memory and visual selection of emotional faces. *Journal of Cognitive Neuroscience, 22*, 1189–1200.

Greicius, M.D., Krasnow, B., Reiss, A.L., & Menon, V. (2003). Functional connectivity in the resting brain: A network analysis of the default mode hypothesis. *Proceedings of the National Academy of Science, 100*(1), 253–258.

Heerema, E. (2021, March 4). White matter in the brain. *Verywellhealth.* https://www.verywellhealth.com/what-is-white-matter-in-the-brain-98119

Hull, K. (2021). Electronic game play therapy. In H.G. Kaduson & C.E. Schaefer (Eds.), *Play therapy with children: Modalities for change* (pp. 55–74). American Psychological Association.

Human Mind (2022). Insula. *Human Mind.* https://human-memory.net/insula/

Jackson, H. (1987). Neural specificity. In G. Adelman (Ed.), *Encyclopedia of neuroscience*, vol II, (pp. 758–760) Birkhäuser.

James, W. (1918). *The principles of psychology, vol. 1–2 (2 volumes in 1).* Pantianos Classics.

MacLean, P.D. (1985). Evolutionary psychiatry and the triune brain. *Psychological Medicine, 15*, 219–221. https://www.cambridge.org/core/services/aop-cambridge-core/content/view/2F0E8159110469F0E85DCD96F032AEB1/S0033291700023485a.pdf/div-class-title-evolutionary-psychiatry-and-the-triune-brain-a-href-fn01-ref-type-fn-span-class-sup-1-span-a-div.pdf

MacLean, P.D. (1970). The triune brain, emotion, and scientific bias. In F.O. Schmit (Ed.), *The neurosciences second study program* (pp. 336–249). Rockefeller University Press.

Medline Plus (n.d.). Myelin. *National Library of Medicine.* https://medlineplus.gov/ency/article/002261.htm

Mohan, A., Roberto, A.J., Mohan, A., Lorenzo, A., Jones, K., Carney, M.J., Loigier-Weyback, L., Hwang, S., & Lapidus, K.A.B. (2016). The significance of the default mode network in neurological and neuropsychiatric disorders: A review. *Yale Journal of Biology and Medicine, 89*, 49–57.

Myers, D.G., & DeWall, C.N. (2018). *Psychology: For the AP course.* Worth.

Oxford Scholarship (2022). Sensory transduction. *University Press Scholarship Online.* https://oxford.universitypressscholarship.com/view/10.1093/oso/9780198835028.001.0001/oso-9780198835028

Padmala, S., Lim, A.L., & Pessoa, L. (2010). Pulvinar and affective significance: Response track moment-to-moment stimulus visibility. *Frontiers in Human Neuroscience, 4*(64), 1–9.

Palay, S.L., & Chan-Palay, V. (1987). Neuron. In G. Adelman (Ed.), *Encyclopedia of neuroscience, vol II* (pp. 812–815). Birkhäuser.

Panksepp, J. (1998). *Affective neuroscience: The foundations of human and animal emotions.* Oxford.

Pressman, P. (2018). Default mode network: The DMN and functional connectivity. *Verywellhealth.* https://www.verywellhealth.com/what-is-the-default-mode-network-2488818

Price, J.L. (1987). Amygdaloid complex. In G. Adelman (Ed.), *Encyclopedia of neuroscience, vol I* (pp. 40–42). Birkhäuser.

Queensland Brain Institute (2017). What are glia? *University of Queensland Australia.* https://qbi.uq.edu.au/brain-basics/brain/brain-physiology/what-are-glia#:~:text=What%20are%20glia%3F%20Glia%20are%20non-neuronal%20cells%20%28i.e.,of%20which%20is%20specialised%20for%20a%20particular%20function

Rafal, R.D., Koller, K., Bultitude, J.H., Mullins, P., Ward, R., Mitchell, A.S., & Bell, A.H. (2014). Connectivity between the superior colliculus and the amygdala in humans and macaque monkeys: Virtual dissection with probabilistic DTI technology. *Journal of Neurophysiology, 114*(3), 1947–1962.

Raichle, M.E. (2015). The brain's default mode network. *Annual Review of Neuroscience, 38,* https://study.com/learn/lesson/cerebral-cortex-function-structure.html433-447

Schmahmann, J.D., Guell, X., Soodley, C.J., & Halko, M.A. (2019). The theory and neuroscience of cerebellar cognition. *Annual Review of Neuroscience, 42,* 337–364. https://pubmed.ncbi.nlm.nih.gov/30939101/

Sciacca, S., Lynch, J., Davagnanam, I., & Barker, R. (2019). Midbrain, pons, and medulla: Anatomy and syndromes. *Radiographics, 39*(4), 1110–1125.

Siegel, D.J. (2012). *Pocket guide to interpersonal biology: An integrative handbook of the mind.* Norton.

Siegel, D.J. (1999). *The developing mind: How relationship and the brain interact to shape who we are.* Guilford.

Stevens, F.L. (2022). *Affective neuroscience in psychotherapy: A clinician's guide for working with emotions.* Routledge.

Tresca, A. (2021). The anatomy of the enteric nervous system. *Verywellhealth.* https://www.verywellhealth.com/enteric-nervous-system-5112820

Van Overwalle, F. (2009). Social cognition and the brain: A meta-analysis. *Human Brain Mapping, 30*(3), 829–858.

Venkatraman, A., Edlow, B.L., & Immordino-Yang, M.H. (2017). The brainstem in emotion: A review. *Frontiers in Neuroanatomy, 11,* 15. https://dash.harvard.edu/bitstream/handle/1/32071942/5343067.pdf?sequence=1

Washmuth, D. (2022, February 16). What is the cerebral cortex? *Study.com.* https://study.com/learn/lesson/cerebral-cortex-function-structure.html

Waxman, S.G. (1987). Axon. In G. Adelman (Ed.), *Encyclopedia of neuroscience, vol I* (pp. 98–101). Birkhäuser.

Worldometer (2022). Current world population. *Worldometer.* http://srv1.worldometers.info/world-population/

Zanto, T.P., & Gazzaley, A. (2013). Fronto-parietal network: Flexible hub of cognitive control. *Trends in Cognitive Sciences, 17*(12), 602–603.

5   Uses, Standards, and Rights

With abstract humankind concepts and behavioral neurobiology concepts explored, we turn to an assortment of the uses, standards, and rights associated with incorporating digital tools in mental health treatment. Moving from the philosophical to the practical, the next few chapters will continue to explore the appropriate therapeutic integration of these tools into our work with clients.

Digital Technology

Use

The statistics regarding the use of digital technology are a bit staggering. On one hand, it is not surprising as we hear about and/or use some type of digital technology daily. If one is older, they can remember the days before the internet, before answering machines; before connection and information were at one's fingertips. There are pros and cons to every development, and the digital technology revolution is no exception. However, what we can say definitively is that it is here to stay for the future.

Digital immigrants, those who were not raised with digital technology but have adopted such technologies into their lives, are typically of the current older generations (Prensky, 2001). Despite having a foot still planted in the past, and perhaps a periodic yearning for the "olden days", digital immigrants are utilizing digital technologies in significant numbers. For instance, 75% of people ages 65 and older use the internet as of a 2021 survey. This is a 24-point increase as compared to the year 2000. Ninety-six percent of people ages 50–64 use the internet as of 2021 (Faverio, 2022). Please refer to Table 5.1 for more age ranges.

DOI: 10.4324/9781003171799-5

Digital natives, however, have fully embraced the use of the internet. A digital native is one who was brought up with digital technologies as a part of life. They have never known life without such advancements (Prensky, 2001). Generation Z, those born between 1995 and 2015, are typically considered digital natives (Perry, 2021). Culture, family values, education, and socioeconomic status certainly impact the members of Generation Z. The year range is more of a timeframe within which the tide shifted and digital natives were born. For people within the Generation Z span of birthyears, ages 18 to 29 in table 8.1, 99% report using the internet as of 2021. The internet is certainly interwoven into our daily lives. There are currently 5.1 billion active users on the internet (Watters, 2022). In the past, legitimate concerns were raised by people who recognized a divide between those who had access and those who did not. The importance revolved around providing services clients could utilize. Thankfully these figures support an increase in internet access and usage and therefore decrease the concerns regarding excluding people in larger numbers Table 5.1.

To have some perspective regarding the magnitude of the incorporations of digital technologies into our lives, here are a few other statistics to consider:

- $705.4 billion (USD) was spent worldwide on information technology devices in 2021
- $491 billion (USD) was spent on enterprise software
- $1.33 trillion (USD) was spent on telecommunication services

Table 5.1 Adapted from "Share of Those 65 and Older Who Are Tech Users Has Grown in the Past Decade," by M. Faverio, 2022, Pew Research, https://www.pewresearch.org/fact-tank/2022/01/13/share-of-those-65-and-older-who-are-tech-users-has-grown-in-the-past-decade/

Age Range	% Who Use The Internet (as of 2021)
18–29 years	99
30–49 years	98
50–64 years	96
65 years and older[*]	75

Notes
[*] In 2000, the gap between the oldest and youngest groups of adults in internet use was 56 percentage points; it now is 24 points.

- 14.91 billion mobile devices in use in 2021; this is projected to grow to 18.22 billion by 2025
- Virtual reality market in 2021 is $4.8 billion (USD) (statista, 2022)

Additionally, CompTIA reports:

- 77% of Americans report having broadband access at home
- More than 90% have internet access
- 4.28 billion users access the internet through their mobile phones
- Social media platforms have 4.2 billion active users
- Wearable technologies are projected to grow globally to include 489.1 million devices by 2023
- $15.7 trillion (USD) is projected to be contributed to the economy by Artificial Intelligence by the year 2030 (Watters, 2022)

Many personal and professional needs are being met through digital tools. We are using hardware and software in education, training, competition, entertainment, travel, medical and mental health treatment, finances, social, lifestyle, utility, productivity, news, and information (Duckma, 2022).

Clinical Fundamentals

Digital play therapy (DPT), digital therapeutics, mHealth, eHealth, computer-mediated psychotherapy (CMP), therapeutic virtual reality (tVR), and VRx are all used to denote some form of clinical/therapeutic digital tool inclusion. The excitement of this is that there is a whole new world of exciting new things to incorporate into the work! However, according to ethical guidelines, clinicians must pursue experience and knowledge within their clinical work.

Per the American Psychological Association (APA), clinicians must uphold the general principles and follow the ethical principles. The APA includes the following in the general principles, which are aspirational: beneficence and nonmaleficence, fidelity and responsibility, integrity, justice, and respect for people's rights and dignity. The ethical principles include: resolving ethical issues, competence, human relations, privacy and confidentiality, advertising and other public statements, record keeping and fees, education and training, research and publication, assessment, and therapy (American Psychological Association, 2016).

Certainly all of the general and ethical principles are important; however, we will highlight a few of the APA principles here for our purpose (2016):

- Beneficence and nonmaleficence – returning to the Hippocratic Oath and Ahimsa, we strive to help those who seek out our services and do no harm.
- Respect for people's rights and dignity – we respect the dignity and worth of all people and protect the vulnerable.
- Competence – practice within one's area of competence; obtain proper training, experience, consultation, and supervision.
- Privacy and confidentiality – maintaining privacy and confidentiality, and any risks to privacy and/or limits to confidentiality shall be discussed.
- Therapy – informed consent shall be discussed and obtained; if utilizing an intervention for which "generally recognized techniques and procedures have not been established, psychologists inform their clients/patients of the developing nature of the treatment, the potential risks involved, alternative treatments that may be available, and the voluntary nature of their participation" (American Psychological Association, 2016, 10:01b).

Customization: Technology Specialists

In 2019, it was suggested that clinics employ "technology specialists". Noel et al., propose that the technology specialist would take an "individualized approach to identify and review electronic resources (e.g., websites, electronic devices, and apps) that may support a client's specific recovery goals (e.g., a sleep cycle-monitoring app or a guided meditation app for someone who wants to improve their sleep)" (2019, p. 59). The technology specialist would be similar to a reference librarian. They would identify relevant hardware and software for a particular client's needs and lay "the groundwork for productive discussions of mental health and technology between clients and members of the clinical team" (pp. 59–60).

Digital Play Therapy

Digital Play Therapy (DPT) arose from the need to define a framework for and structure within what was recognized as a powerful therapeutic intervention: the use of digital play in therapy (Stone, 2019, 2022). The intention of this modality is to provide clinicians an assortment of ways to interact with their clients utilizing tools that were either (a) known to the client; a part of their world or (b) unknown to the client; but with therapeutic properties identified by the clinician. The intention of the framework and structure was to ensure that the ethical and general principles were integrated. Please refer to the text, *Digital Play Therapy, 2nd edition* for more detailed information (Stone, 2022).

Applying concepts from the APA principles and expanding upon them, DPT includes the 5Cs: Competency, Culture, Comfort, Congruence, and Capability. These principles are included to alert the clinician to the importance of knowing what one is doing and why they are doing it, along with striving toward all 5Cs in the treatments provided.

Competency

Competency requires that the clinician possesses "the quality or state of having sufficient knowledge, judgment, skill, or strength (as for a particular duty or in a particular respect)" and "the knowledge that enables a person to speak and understand a language" (Merriam-Webster, 2019, para. 1). Clinicians must "obtain, maintain, and exhibit solid clinical skills, knowledge, and judgement" (Stone, 2022, p. 30). Through research, education, experience, consultation, and supervision, a clinician can aspire to high levels of knowledge, integrity, and professionalism (Stone, 2022).

Culture

"Culture is the characteristics and knowledge of a particular group of people, encompassing language, religion, cuisine, social habits, music and arts" (McKelvie & Pappas, 2021, para. 1). We strive to respect, honor, explore, and acknowledge cultural diversity and humility. For our purposes, we want to include the traditional understandings of culture, along with the inclusion of a person's identification and representation, including their interest in and use of digital tools. "Subjective experiences such as age, gender, sexual orientation, dis (ability), socioeconomic status, generation, marital status, interests, education, occupation, hobbies etc., should also be considered when discussing culture and diversity" (Jiminez-Pride, 2022, p. 68).

Comfort and Congruence

Internal comfort is often palpable to others. Knowledge, a solid sense of self, and confidence in one's knowledge base permeates through our interactions with our clients. Coming to a clinician for guidance and assistance, the client will benefit from interactions with a clinician who is comfortable with their knowledge base. Comfort is achieved through obtaining and integrating experience and knowledge.

Congruence is attained, within this purpose, when the clinician is able to

> *attend to, and be in as much agreement as possible with, their own biases, attitudes, opinions, and desires. The balance needs to happen between the therapist's own comfort and belief systems and the needs of the client. If these are incongruent, the relationship between the therapist and client, and therefore the therapeutic process, will be negatively affected.*
>
> (Stone, 2022, p. 34)

Achieving comfort and congruence is traditionally achieved through education, consultation, and supervision. Each of these, along with research and experience, will assist the therapist with achieving a new level of comfort and congruence when an incongruence is recognized (Stone, 2022).

Three Levels of DPT

Recognizing that there a number of variables involved in the decision to incorporate digital tools into mental health services, digital play therapy can be used in any of three defined levels, or a combination within sessions or across treatment. The level used will be determined by the treatment goals and plan, client interest and comfort, and therapist knowledge and 5Cs.

> Level 1: Any inclusion of the client's digital tool interests in the session. This can be simply an open acceptance of the inclusion of the client discussing their experiences, interests, queries, etc., regarding their own use. This includes hardware and software, videos, social media, readings, vloggers, and more. The client is invited and encouraged to share this portion of their life with the clinician. Level 1 does not include any devices; rather, it is the verbal and nonverbal sharing and discussion of these topics.
>
> Level 2: In addition to the components of level 1, level 2 includes the inclusion of the hardware and software they would like to share. This includes using a device and/or program/app and

sharing, exploring, and watching together. One could look up song lyrics, watch a video, research information, or showing a particular game. The client and clinician do not engage in direct play together, rather it is focused on sharing and observing that which is of interest to the client on a digital device.

Level 3: Level 3 includes everything from levels 1 and 2 plus the engagement in direct play together on a digital device. Using a single or multiplayer program together is an example of DPT level 3 engagement. The play is interpreted and analyzed according to the clinician's theoretical foundation.

*adapted from Digital Play Therapy, 2nd ed.,
by J. Stone, 2022, Routledge

Clients of all ages are utilizing digital tools in their day-to-day lives. Those who are "gaming" are included in a 2021 $178.2 billion industry. In 2022, it is expected to reach $196 billion, and it will continue to increase thereafter (Hadji-Vasilev, 2022; Stone, 2022). About 81% of Generation Z, 77% of Millennials, 60% of Generation X, and 42% of Baby Boomers play video games. When asked how playing games affects them, 90% state gaming brings them joy, 87% mental stimulation, 87% stress relief, 81% teamwork skills, and 79% inspiration. These are not only children playing, either. The percentages of Americans who play video games include 67% adults and 76% children (Hadji-Vasilev, 2022).

Regardless of our personal opinions regarding these numbers, there is a very high chance that some type of digital hardware and software is being used by our clients, no matter the age. Over time, these numbers will certainly increase as Generation Z grows older and the next generations of digital natives are born. For many, it is clinically, culturally, and ethically appropriate to incorporate digital tools into mental health treatment; it is the language of many.

Digital Therapeutics

Digital Therapeutics (DTx) is described as a "health discipline and treatment option that utilizes a digital and often online health technologies to treat a medical or psychological condition" (Digital Health London, 2018, p. 3). The Digital Therapeutics Alliance states: "Digital therapeutics (DTx) deliver evidence-based therapeutic interventions that are driven by high quality software programs to prevent, manage, or treat a medical disorder or disease" (2019a, para 1).

Table 5.2 Digital Therapeutics Alliance Foundational Principles (Digital Therapeutics Alliance, 2019a, para 4)

1 Prevent, manage, or treat a medical disorder or disease
2 Produce a medical intervention that is driven by software
3 Incorporate design, manufacture, and quality best practices
4 Engage end users in product development and usability processes
5 Incorporate patient privacy and security protections
6 Apply product deployment, management, and maintenance best practices
7 Publish trial results inclusive of clinically-meaningful outcomes in peer-reviewed journals
8 Be reviewed and cleared or certified by regulatory bodies as required to support product claims of risk, efficacy, and intended use
9 Make claims appropriate to clinical evaluation and regulatory status
10 Collect, analyze, and apply real-world evidence and/or product performance data

Used alone or in conjunction with other treatments, DTx "products incorporate advanced technology best practices relating to design, clinical evaluation, usability, and data security" (para 2).

The Digital Therapeutics Alliance states that any products which claim to be a digital therapeutic must adhere to the following (Table 5.2).

They have also created a code of ethics regarding the digital therapeutic products. Familiarizing oneself with these details serves multiple purposes: (1) there are organizations attending to the structure of such tools, (2) understand that organizations are creating frameworks and standards for such tools to protect clients, (3) some of these standards and principles can be applied to other digital tools, not just formal digital therapeutics, and (4) these standards (and others) can inform the creation of other standards.

The Digital Therapeutics Industry Code of Ethics aims to "establishe<s> principles to which every company engaged in the design, evaluation, and deployment of digital therapeutics1 should adhere" (Digital Therapeutics Alliance, 2019b, para 1).

1 Demonstrate a commitment to patient safety. Do no harm.
2 Develop interventions that improve the quality of care, clinical outcomes, and quality of life.
3 Protect patients' rights to privacy, consent, and knowledge of data use.
4 Directly align the product definition, claims, benefits, and risks with all analytical and clinical evaluation outcomes.
5 Make claims appropriate to product status within each applicable regulatory jurisdiction.

6 Ensure that credible evidence supporting product claims and outcomes is readily available to patients, caregivers, clinicians, and payors.
7 Bring products to market in a responsible way.
8 Verify that products perform as expected and deliver on stated claims
9 Ensure that product security, data, and functionality are not compromised.
10 Maintain a culture of quality and organizational excellence (para 2).

World Health Organization

The 139th and 142nd sessions of the World Health Organization created a report regarding the "use of appropriate digital technologies for public health was held in May of 2016". The purpose of this report was to address the use of digital technologies for public health in an effort to provide "cost-effective and secure use of information and communication technologies in support of health and health-related fields" (World Health Organization, 2018, para 3).

The report acknowledged that digital technologies were becoming an important resource for the delivery of health services. At the time, they recognized mobile devices as "particularly relevant, due to their ease of use, broad reach, and wide acceptance" and quoted that over 70% of the world's mobile phones in 2015 were in low-middle-income countries (World Health Organization, 2018, para 4).

The World Bank Group stated that mobile phones were the "most ubiquitous modern technology: in some developing countries, more people have access to a mobile phone than to a bank account, electricity, or even clean water" (World Bank Group, 2012, para 1). Due to the ubiquitousness of mobile devices, they have been found to be powerful tools with people who have serious mental illness (Ben-Zeev et al., 2018; Firth et al., 2015; Halverson et al., 2022; Batra et al., 2017; Beard et al., 2019).

The spread of digital technologies and global interconnectedness has a significant potential to accelerate Member States' progress towards achieving universal health coverage, including ensuring access to quality health services. Increasing the capacity of Member States to implement digital health, and in particular mHealth, could play a major role in realizing that potential, particularly:

1 *By increasing access to quality health services*
2 *by increasing access to sexual and reproductive health services;*
3 *by reducing maternal, child and neonatal mortality.*

4   *by reducing premature mortality from noncommunicable diseases and noncommunicable disease comorbidities*

5   *by increasing global health security. by increasing the safety and quality of care*

6   *by increasing patient, family, and community engagement.* (World Health Organization, 2018, pp. 3–4)

Neuro-rights

"Technological advancements are redefining human life and are transforming the role of humans in society. In particular, neuro-technology – or methods to record, interpret, or alter brain activity – has the potential to profoundly alter what it means to be human" (Yuste et al., 2021, p. 154). As discussed in the behavioral neuroscience chapter, the brain is an intricate, interconnected, complex organ capable of sending messages regarding cognition, learning, emotion, memory, imagination, behavior, movement, and more throughout the brain, mind, and body. Technologies have advanced in amazing ways; with the ability to interpret, monitor, and collect biodata we can learn more about humans and lead to significant scientific and medical breakthroughs (Yuste et al., 2021). However, this also creates ways that the information can be used for marketing, tracking, and "unprecedented human rights implications" (Yuste et al., 2021, p. 155).

Neurotechnology is being developed worldwide in ways that will lead to new treatments for neurological diseases and mental illness, such as Alzheimer's, stroke, post-traumatic stress disorder, schizophrenia, addiction, and depression (Yuste et al., 2021). The more information we have about etiologies and processes, the better we can know when, how, and where to intervene for the health of the client. To perform due diligence, we must learn more to understand how something works to fully assess the advancement in question.

With any new advancement comes considerations. It is our responsibility, particularly as clinicians, to explore and assess new advancements so that we may protect the client and ensure informed consent is as thorough as possible. Neurotechnology includes brain-computer interfaces or BCIs. BCIs connect a brain to a computer and allow bidirectional communication between the outside world and the brain through either a helmet (noninvasive) or a unit inside a person's head (invasive). This allows information from the brain to be exported to a data base and the brain activity to be altered (Yuste et al., 2021).

There are many questions which arise regarding the use of such technology. Some of them are very positive; the possibilities to help people with psychological and medical difficulties are exciting and invigorating! However, one question which has arisen is regarding neuro-rights – who owns a person's neuroinformation or neurodata? Yuste et al. posed this concern in their article entitled *It's Time for Neuro-Rights: New Human Rights for the Age of Neurotechnology*. They highlight the gap in human rights protections, which historically have not had to be concerned with neurodata. The need for guidelines, principles, and policies was introduced, particularly because this technology "directly interacts with and affects the brain" (2021, p. 159). Historically one's brain activity was their own, contained within their own brain, secured from others unless intentionally shared. Now questions regarding free will and private thoughts arise, with the "presumption of mental privacy" brought into question (p. 159).

As the behavioral neuroscience chapter discussed, there are millions of messages transmitted throughout the brain without the conscious knowledge of the person. If the neurotechnology can translate those messages into neurodata, the person could be relaying unknown and unintentional information. How can we protect such data? The International Covenant on Civil and Political Rights (ICCPR) is a treaty which has been adopted by 173 countries and protects more than 90% of the world's population. Typically it protects humans from racial discrimination, rights of women, children, and people with disabilities, disappearances, and torture. In the age of neurotechnolgy, Yuste et al. propose neuro-rights be included within the ICCPR's Article 17, the prohibition of "unlawful or arbitrary interferences with privacy" (p. 160).

The proposed neuro-rights are:

1   *the right to identity, or the ability to control both one's physical and mental integrity*
2   *the right to agency, or the freedom of thought and free will to choose one's own actions*
3   *the right to mental privacy, or the ability to keep thoughts protected against disclosure*
4   *the right to fair access to mental augmentation, or the ability to ensure that the benefits of improvements to sensory and mental capacity through neurotechnology are distributed justly in the population*
5   *the right to protection from algorithmic bias, or the ability to ensure that technologies do not insert prejudices* (Yuste et al., 2021, pp. 160–161).

The right to "cognitive liberty" and the right to "mental privacy" are central to the concerns about neuro-rights (Global Neuroethics, n.d.). The call for countries to enact neuro-rights is being raised by a number of individuals and groups, however, to date Chile is the only country who has enacted legislation (Moody, 2021; Zúñiga-Fajuri, 2021).

One of the key differences between personal and professional use of digital technologies is the need to evaluate the use with a focus on thoughtful, thorough, multidimensional analysis. Keeping one's professional ethics at the forefront, how can technologies be used for the good of humanity and how can humanity be protected from those who might do harm?

References

American Psychological Association (2016). Ethical principles of psychologists and code of conduct. *American Psychiatric Association.*

Batra, S., Baker, R.A., Wang, T., Forma, F.; DiBiasi, F., & Peters-Strickland, T. (2017). Digital health technology for use in patients with serious mental health illness: A systematic review of the literature. *Medical Devices: Evidence and Research, 10*, 237–251.

Beard, C., Silverman, A.L., Foregeard, M., Wilmer, M.T., Torous, J., & Björgvinisson, T. (2019). Smartphone, social media, and mental health app use in an acute transdiagnostic psychiatric sample. *JMIT Mhealth and Uhealth, 7*(6), 1–12. https://pubmed.ncbi.nlm.nih.gov/31199338/

Ben-Zeev, D., Brian, R.M., Jonathan, G., Razzano, L., Pashka, N., Carpenter-Song, E., Drake, R.E., & Scherer, E.A. (2018). Mobile health (mHealth) versus clinic-based group intervention for people with serious mental illness: A randomized controlled trial. *Psychiatric Services, 69*(9), 978–985.

Digital Health London (2018). Digital therapeutics in the NHS: The rise of digital therapies & the evidence that proves they work. *Digital Health London.* https://digitalhealth.london/wp-content/uploads/2018/04/DigitalTherapeuticsNHS.pdf

Digital Therapeutics Alliance (2019a). Digital therapeutics definition and core principles. *Digital Therapeutics Alliance.* https://dtxalliance.org/wp-content/uploads/2021/01/DTA_DTx-Definition-and-Core-Principles.pdf

Digital Therapeutics Alliance (2019b). DTx industry code of ethics. *Digital Therapeutics Alliance* https://dtxalliance.org/wp-content/uploads/2021/01/DTA_DTx-Industry-Code-of-Ethics_11.11.19.pdf

Duckma (2022). *What are the different types of mobile apps? Breaking down industries and functionalities.* Duckma. https://blog.duckma.com/en/types-of-mobile-apps/

Faverio, M. (2022). Share of those 65 and older who are tech users has grown in the past decade. *Pew Research.* https://www.pewresearch.org/fact-tank/2022/01/13/share-of-those-65-and-older-who-are-tech-users-has-grown-in-the-past-decade/

Firth, J., Cotter, J., Torous, J., Bucci, S., Firth, J.A., & Yung, A.R. (2015). Mobile phone ownership and endorsement of mHealth" among people with psychosis: A meta-analysis of cross-sectional studies. *Schizophrenia Bulletin.* https://pubmed.ncbi.nlm.nih.gov/26400871/

Global Neuroethics (n.d.). Neurorights. *Global Neuroethics.* https://globalneuro ethics.com/neurorights/

Hadji-Vasilev, A. (2022). 23 video game and online gaming statistics, facts, and trends for 2022. *Cloudwards.* https://www.cloudwards.net/online-gaming-statistics/

Halverson, T.F., Browne, J., Thomas, S.M., & Palenski, P. (2022). An examination of neurocognition and theory of mind as predictors of engagement with a tailored digital therapeutic in persons with serious mental illness. *Schizophrenia Research, 28,* 1–9. https://www.sciencedirect.com/science/article/pii/S2215001322000014?ref=pdf_download&fr=RR-2&rr=71729e511cbcb49f

Jiminez-Pride, C. (2022). Cultural humility in the telehealth playroom. In J. Stone (Ed.), *Play therapy and telemental health: Foundations, populations, & interventions* (pp. 68–83). Routledge.

Lagan, S., Sandler, L., & Torous, J. (2021). Evaluating evaluation frameworks: A scoping review of frameworks for assessing health apps. *BMJ Open, 11,* 1–8. https://www.ncbi.nlm.nih.gov/pmc/articles/PMC7986656/

McKelvie, C. & Pappas, S. (2021, December 15). What is culture? *Live Science.* https://www.livescience.com/21478-what-is-culture-definition-of-culture.html

Merriam Webster (2019, August). *Competence.* www.merriam-webster.com/dictionary/competence

Moody, G. (2021, August 25). Chile is passing a neuro-rights law to protect mental privacy. It's time for other nations to do the same. *PIABlog.* https://www.privateinternetaccess.com/blog/chile-is-passing-a-neuro-rights-law-to-protect-mental-privacy-its-time-for-other-nations-to-do-the-same/

Noel, V.A., Carpenter-Song, E., Acquilano, S.C., Torous, J., & Drake, R.E. (2019). A technology specialist: A 21st century support role in clinical care. *Nature Partner Journal Digital Medicine, 2*(61), 59–61. https://www.nature.com/articles/s41746-019-0137-6

Perry, D. (2021, April 13). Everything you need to know about the new generation Z. *Revenues and Profits.* https://revenuesandprofits.com/digital-natives/

Prensky, M. (2001). Digital natives digital immigrants. *On The Horizon (MCB Univeristy Press), 9*(5), 1–6. https://www.marcprensky.com/writing/Prensky%20-%20Digital%20Natives,%20Digital%20Immigrants%20-%20Part1.pdf

Statista (2022). Technology and telecommunications. *Statista.* https://www.statista.com/markets/418/technology-telecommunications/

Stone, J. (2022). *Digital play therapy: The clinician's guide to comfort and competence*, 2nd ed. Routledge.

Stone, J. (2019). *Digital play therapy: The clinician's guide to comfort and competence*. Routledge.

Watters, A. (2022, February 3). 25 crucial information technology statistics & facts to know. *CompTIA*. https://connect.comptia.org/blog/information-technology-stats-facts

World Bank (2012). Information and communications for development: Maximizing mobile. *Open Knowledge Repository*. https://openknowledge.worldbank.org/handle/10986/11958

World Health Organization (2018, March 26). mHealth: Use of appropriate digital technologies for public health. *Seventy-first World Health Assembly, Provisional Agenda Item 12.4*. https://apps.who.int/gb/ebwha/pdf_files/WHA71/A71_20-en.pdf

Yuste, R., Genser, J., & Herrmann, S. (2021). It's time for neuro-rights: New human rights for the age of neurotechnology. *Horizons, 18*, 154–164. https://www.cirsd.org/en/horizons/horizons-winter-2021-issue-no-18/its-time-for-neuro--rights

Zúñiga-Fajuri, A., Miranda, L.V., Miralles, D.Z., & Venegas, R.S. (2021). Neurorights in Chile: Between neuroscience and legal science. *Developments in Neuroethics and Bioethics, 4*, 165–179.

6 Clinical Concepts

This is where it all comes together. We have discussed the fundamentals; the abstract concepts which we must evaluate in our interactions, communications, and cognitive processes. We have explored the brain and its functions; the process by which emotions, memories, cognition, and learning occur and are processed, organized, and stored. Let us discuss the overview and then apply the concepts to the process and experience of using digital tools in therapy.

This chapter intends to highlight a number of key concepts within each of the previous two chapters (Fundamental Concepts and Behavioral Neuroscience) and briefly integrate them with the ways digital play therapy either activates, addresses, or incorporates each into therapeutic work. The clinician can further these conceptualizations based on their theoretical foundation and beliefs surrounding the activation of change within the client. All other clinical processes apply, i.e., ethics, standards, and protections, as the use of digital tools in therapy, or digital play therapy (DPT), is a modality and should be incorporated as such.

Concepts

How we see ourselves, in representation, perception, role, and identity contributes to the realization that we exist as a distinct being from others.

How we represent ourselves in during therapeutic digital play, or digital play therapy (DPT), is a reflection of either how we feel or are, how we have felt or been, or how we would like to feel or be. This representation is both visual in how a character or avatar is depicted and in what kind of behavior is exhibited during the game play. The clinician can understand more about what is important to the client regarding identification and representation based upon the client's chosen depiction.

DOI: 10.4324/9781003171799-6

Self-awareness progresses developmentally from confusion to differentiation, situation to identification, permanence to self-consciousness, to lead us toward a recognition of how we may be represented in our minds and the minds of others.

Depending upon the stage of one's self-awareness progression, one might be struggling with self-awareness, boundaries, and self-perception. How we see ourselves and understand our place in the world can be projected onto our character/avatar within a game during DPT. Approaches to the play and interactions can alert the clinician to the client's self-awareness developmental level and how that might impact the client's day-to-day life.

Interoception includes our ability to interpret our internal states of sensing, integrating, and regulating self and emotions through the interplay between the autonomic and central nervous systems, and contributes toward emotional experiences, feelings, and decision-making. Consciousness, having been represented to the self, includes the known perceptions which originate from within the body and the understandings from the mind.

The direction of the information being communicated: from inside the body or from outside the body; from the body to the brain or the brain to the body, informs us about the stimuli that the client is attending to and receiving information from. We will certainly not be able to determine the nervous system components within a session, but it is important to conceptualize the possible origins of information, where and how it travels, and what the impact might be on the client.

Consciously connecting with our bodily cues and sensations provides a deeper level of awareness of self, cause and effect, the impact of emotions on the body (somatic responses), and a deeper understanding of our decisions. Within DPT, a clinician can perceive, interpret, and discuss these connections with the client periodically throughout the play, i.e., "When that troll attacked you, how did you experience it? Where did you feel it in your body? How did your breathing change? Your heartrate?", etc.

Our level of consciousness impacts every aspect of our internal process, interactions with others, and behavior. Through DPT, the clinician and client work together to bring important aspects of approaches and perceptions to a new level of consciousness. This can be achieved through discussion, reflection, and recognition of emerging and/or existing response patterns exhibited during the play interactions.

Introspection is the mechanism by which we look inward to examine and evaluate our thoughts and feelings.

Perceptions combine our prior understandings and experiences with sensory input, observations, and memories to form a more comprehensive cognition.

Theory of mind includes the recognition and anticipation that we and others have internal states; we attempt to attribute qualities to those internal states, and we realize that such states may not be clear. Recognition of thought, feeling, needs, and desire for self and others allows for a potential reciprocal interaction.

Self-reflections regarding our cognitions, emotions, and behaviors allow us to understand more about ourselves and our experiences. Introspection within DPT can include both the client's internal process and realizations during the game play and the interpretations and reflections provided by the clinician.

Bringing one's perceptions to consciousness, discussing and/or experiencing the process of integrating sensory input, observations, and memories into meaning, and culminating that into a further understanding and pattern changes can result in significant growth for the client. Through the use of DPT, the observations, discussions, interactions, and interventions allow the client and clinician to support or challenge the client's perceptions.

The recognition of self and other, as well as the realization that internal states can fluctuate, are important component of social interaction and the establishment of self-worth, other-worth, and relational experiences. Within DPT, the clinician can assist the client with theory of mind-oriented realizations, empathy, sympathy, and recognition of the feeling and needs of self and other. Through the process, an exploration of appropriate boundary setting can occur, as well as discussion of responses when one's boundaries are violated.

Other can be realized once the self is recognized; the perception and understanding of other allows for a separation from the self. Self-other recognizes that the relationship between self and other is bidirectional, with the psychological influence toward each potentially unknown, but accounted for. Double consciousness addresses the concept of looking at one's self through the eyes of others, with a comparison of self-concept and other's-concept, and acknowledgment of the potential impact of all.

DPT interactions can be subtle or overt depending on the software used. One can play games with quests to achieve toward the needs of the self, other, or group. Expressive creations can be completed to depict self, other, relational experiences, and the establishment of personal boundaries. The possibilities are virtually endless. The recognition of self and others allows for the acknowledgment of needs; the realizations that one's needs may be similar or different than others' and/or the exploration of getting those needs met or meeting those of others. Identification of needs can lead to the exploration of resources, allocation, and assignment of such resources, multitask sequencing, and concepts of self-preservation.

The bidirectional qualities within self-other and double consciousness allow for the recognition and inclusion of how people impact each other in interactions or even in existence or absence. The exploration of the psychological influence of each allows one to further understand the complex impacts occurring within and around a person. Understanding these impacts allows the clinician and client to identify areas which could benefit from change to improve areas of difficulty. DPT, and the ability for interaction between clinician and client and client and others, provides ample opportunities for these interactions to occur and therapeutic interventions to be implemented.

In-group identification refers to the ways we self-identify within a group dynamic and whether or not the self-identification is stable or variable depending upon the environment. Relational selves include the varied representation of self as it is dependent upon the relationships with others and the potential mental health impacts of a self-identity which has greater variability.

Through a variety of environments and perspectives, relationships bring two or more people together to form connections, and hopefully a community, so the participants can benefit in ways that impact all parties; how people see themselves, each other, and their worlds have reciprocal impacts on the health and well-being of all participants.

DPT is particularly well suited for therapeutic work that includes in-group identification and the understanding of relational selves. There are vast approaches and opportunities available in the digital space, offered through a range of characters, representations, and scenarios. The exploration of each within team or group game play, without day-to-day life consequences, particularly within a clinical relationship, allows for complex and powerful therapeutic interactions.

Regulating the flow of energy and information, the mind includes being conscious and aware, experiencing emotion, thinking, and memories, and is interdependent with subjective experiences, information, and relationships which impact the body and potentially the structure of the brain. Continuing to learn about the self, brain, mind, and body are imperative to continuing to understand the ways we can access and assist our clients with their psychological difficulties.

Immersion is an engagement within an absorptive, flow-like state and experience. Immersive experiences can transcend the physical reality, whether internally or externally, dependent upon the environment and stimuli, to create an absorptive experience.

The brain and body are impacted by the flow of energy and connection within the entire body. When the flow of energy and experiences of emotion, thought, and memories are dysregulated, a person is unable to properly assess and react to stimuli and situations. DPT engagement allows for a wide variety of experiences within which to identify response patterns and bring them into consciousness. The clinician and client can then explore and identify alternate ways to integrate emotion, thought, memories, experiences, information, and relationships with healthier conceptualizations and responses for generalization to an improved day-to-day life.

DPT immersion allows the client to truly embody and experience the environment and stimulus for the exploration of self, other, perception, interoception, integration, identity, representation, and purpose. This allows for the adjustment of responses as well as the ability to practice such adjustments within a safe environment. There is minimal direct, in-the-moment impact on the client's day-to-day life, but significant impacts are possible once the new knowledge is applied to future interactions and experiences.

Neuroplasticity refers to the brain's ability to adapt in both functional and structural ways, with much to learn and enormous implications for psychological treatment, interventions, and understandings.

The ability to functionally adjust and adapt requires plasticity of the brain and mind. Understanding that change can happen on physical, emotional, and behavioral levels supports the therapeutic process entirely. DPT allows for situations to be witnessed by the clinician in client-chosen activities and intentionally incorporated by the clinician when clinician-chosen. The response to a series of similar stimuli allows the clinician recognize patterns which most likely impact the client's relationships and behaviors outside of the therapeutic environment. Understanding these patterns and themes with more depth informs and expands the therapeutic relationship and process.

Purpose is the reason something exists; intention is an aim or purpose which serves as determination to act. Together, purpose and intention drive us toward meaningful behavior, planning, and understanding toward meaning and reason. That which exists has substance and can be objectively perceived, whether they are independent or dependent, real or functional. Reality can be in the "eye of the beholder"; of subjective or objective qualities to exist due to substance or a creator, and dependent upon perception.

Purpose and reality can be extended to self, other, and object. People who engage in digital play conceptualize the stimuli as having purpose and existing, particularly within the interrelated environment of a game. The resource which is gathered to further a goal has purpose and reality to it as it is used intentionally within the game play. The purpose and reality extend to the perception of self, other, and object in terms of perceived value in the interaction. This is particularly powerful and relevant in the therapeutic setting; even if the clinician is not aware of the purpose, an important component of therapy is to uncover and process that which is purposeful for our clients.

Presence and telepresence are distinguished primarily by the environment; both are psychological states or subjective perceptions; however, one is in the physical presence and one is generated by or filtered through human made technology.

The conceptualization of embodiment is a complex, abstract construct intertwined with self-concept and perception, whereby the immediate sensations and stored representations influence one's embodiment perceptions.

The sense of presence, for the self and/or other, can impact the client in a number of ways. The presence of another can be comforting or disturbing, depending on the situation and history of the client. Experiencing presence and telepresence within DPT allows the clinician and client to process any reactions elicited by the game play. The mind and body can perceive one's own presence and the presence of others in an environment and interact as though it were happening in their physical space and existence. There can be a self-other quality to the interaction, in that the client can experience what it means to them to be present within the environment, where the self and other are distinct, and where they might intertwine or join. These explorations can be philosophical, relational, and physical, particularly when paired with embodiment.

Proprioception allows us to navigate through a variety of environments and spaces via a biological process whereby information is relayed throughout the body and processed by the brain for coordinated movement, gait, and posture.

The nervous systems impact critical responses in the body, whether it be transporting information to or from the brain. The information that is communicated, processed, and then acted upon within this complex system impacts our safety, arousal, memory, learning, cognition, pleasure, movement, and behavior.

The DMN and CEN are particularly salient when conceptualizing the process of the brain which works to achieve internal balance. We strive to understand emotions, perceptions, and behaviors and these networks contribute to the abilities of the body to experience homeostasis.

DPT which includes movement, particularly virtual reality, allows for a higher level of coordinated body awareness, as well as activation of many parts of the brain. The sympathetic and parasympathetic systems and the DMN and CEN networks relay and process information which can impact conceptualizations and behavior, which in turn, impact the sense of self, boundaries, and relationships.

Play is a critical component of human nature and development across the lifespan; identification of the expressed or demonstrated components of play allows a view into the world of the player, through the demonstration of enjoyable little worlds. Both pretence and quarantining are important components of play; the ability to employ representational, meta-representational, mentalistic, cognitive, and theory of mind concepts to play, while maintaining the ability to quarantine, allows for free play assignment, expression, and creation.

DPT is centered around play, whatever the age of the client. A therapist who observes and engages in play with a client is able to witness and further understand the client's world and worldview; how the client sees the world and themselves in it; how people are treated and how one will accept being treated. Through play, once can suspend day-to-day life through pretense and further explore the dynamics impacting their lives. The ability to quarantine, developed at an early age, allows once to appropriately separate reality from pretense. The clinician guides which items and concepts would benefit the client to be removed from quarantine and integrated into cognitions, and DPT allows for the practice of this integration.

The hypothalamus, amygdala, thalamus, and hippocampus serve many purposes within the human brain: memory, motivation, and learning, response, regulation, attachment, behavior, and attention. Continuing to explore not only the structural components of the brain through improving technologies, but also expanding our understanding of the human experience and process while applying the learning to psychological concepts and approaches will improve the care we provide.

The activation of the hypothalamus, amygdala, thalamus, and hippocampus sparks a cascade of information relays and processing of stimuli which stimulates pathways throughout the brain and body. Visual and auditory stimuli are of particular interest in this arena, as well as stored memories and neural nets. Access to these areas within a clinical setting allows for supported processing and reorganization of experiences, responses, and belief systems.

DPT experiences can allow a person to customize themselves and/or an environment for the processing and reorganization to occur. One's approach to the play and perceptions of the scenarios within inform the exploration and expression of memory, motivation, learning, response, regulation, attachment, behavior, and attention. The clinician is able to witness and conceptualize the client's worldview.

Historically people have believed that it is digital game play that creates something, i.e., depression, anxiety, violence, etc. Perhaps it is the opposite, that digital game play, and by extension DPT, engages the hypothalamus, amygdala, thalamus, and hippocampus through visual and auditory stimuli and allows the brain, mind, and body to access the memories, motivations, learnings, and responses and informing us of their abilities for regulation, attachment, behavior, and attention. It is a pathway which allows access to many interconnected processes and components, including concerning symptoms, and not a creation of the symptoms and/or ensuing responses. This is an important area for future exploration. The hypothesis is that we are able to access more of this information through digital play and in DPT we are able to fold that information into the treatment plan and clinical work.

The superior and inferior colliculi process visual and auditory signals prior to being transmitted to other portions of the brain; what we attend to, what we preliminarily perceive as scary and/or threatening, is decided on, in part, by these structures. These decisions impact our actions and reactions, and depending on the perceived level of danger, may or may not initially involve the frontal lobe.

Visual and auditory stimuli inform the person of the environment and whether actions or reactions must occur. DPT provides a plethora of visual and auditory input to be processed and responded to, which the clinician can observe and witness. The clinician attends with the intention of processing and/or intervening as warranted.

In psychotherapeutic work, it may behoove us to expose clients to a predefined level of perceived threat so we can pause mid process to encourage and guide toward the higher order processing of the situation.

Cognition and metacognition are enormous, abstract concepts which engage multiple brain structures to process information and sensations, connect them with emotions and memories, and can result in thoughts and/or actions. Cognition can be thought of as thinking, and metacognition as thinking about thinking.

Experiences populate our memories, inform our cognitions and decision-making; they are the building blocks which construct many aspects of who we might become, who we are, and how we move through our lives.

In DPT, we are employing cognition and metacognition, as well as many other processes, in an effort to engage emotions, thoughts, memories, and actions. Through representative game play, we can explore a person's thought process to understand a task or goal, the process and strategy to meet these, and the execution abilities of the client. The process witnessed within DPT is most likely paralleled within their interactions outside of the clinical session. The clinician conceptualizes these components in relation to the knowledge about the client and creates parallels so the newly understood information can be integrated.

Identification and representation of the self to ourselves and others impacts how we feel about ourselves, the world, and our place within it; to honor and respect one's self can lead to truth and knowing; self-acceptance and identity; purposeful steps toward self-actualization.

Identification and representation are key aspects of every concept within this chapter. How we identify and represent ourselves impacts our self, others, self-other, and our in-group perceptions, which, in turn, activates many brain structures and networks. Ultimately, this influences and shapes our reality. DPT allows the client to explore the concepts of identity and representation in the ways they or the clinician might find to be necessary for growth. One can explore a variety of ways of being in a trial-and-error approach to safely identifying that which is meaningful to the client. The guidance of the clinician can help the client feel safe and supported throughout this process.

The brain is believed to have areas of higher cortical and cognitive functioning, and those which are more primitive. However, the areas are interconnected and we continue to learn more about the functions and relationship of all the areas. Although the brain has been defined in terms of regions, it is a highly interconnected organ whose impact reaches throughout via dendritic connections. Conceptualizing the brain in more of a systems perspective than individualistic is important for psychological work.

As we continue to learn more about the brain, mind, and body, our clinical work will grow in terms of connectivity and depth; to further understand the human being and their existence in this physical world and in their representational worlds. We continue toward the knowledge of self and other and of connectedness and independence – and the many systems impacted by all. It is the way of the brain, the body, the earth, and existence, and the use of digital tools speaks to aspects of each. Continuing to understand more propels us toward our lifelong journey of capability and possibility.

Clinical Populations

Digital Play Therapy can be used with a variety of clients. First and foremost, if the use of digital tools is of interest to a client, then it will be important to invite the incorporation. The client's age is of less importance, as hardware and software is available for all age groups. For younger clients, discussions with caregivers and explicit informed consent will be critical components of care. Within DPT, there are clinical decisions which can (and should) be made to tailor the experience to the needs of the client, whatever the age, diagnosis, or needs.

Digital play therapy can be incorporated in many settings and environments, including but not limited to private practice, agencies, schools, hospitals, and crisis environments. The vast variety of options available allows the clinician to customize the experience to the specific clinical needs of the client, which expands the reach of this amazing modality.

Additional Concepts Within Gameplay

We can identify a number of therapeutic factors included in digital game play.

For example: strategy, frustration tolerance, taking care of self, finding, accessing, and utilizing resources, nurturing the therapeutic powers of play, team building, trial-and-error, multisequential tasks, social skills, competition, identification, perception, introspection, representation, self, other, self-awareness, consciousness, introspection, theory of mind, other, self-other, double consciousness, in-group identification and relational selves, boundaries, coping skills, and more. Due to the vast options, as mentioned earlier, the informed clinician can choose programs to use within session that will benefit the client through their unique therapeutic process.

Moving Forward with Digital Tools

Humans will continue to define and redefine the needs and uses of digital tools, along with the difficulties, that arise over the upcoming generations. Boundaries will be placed and challenged. Ultimately, it is typically that which adds value which withstands the test of time.

The pendulum will swing, from technopanic to widespread adoption, and then will settle into balance – until the next upheaval (Stone, 2019; 2022). These are the physics of our lives; the pendulum bob is first displaced from its equilibrium and released. It swings in periodic motion, back and forth in a regular and repeating manner, only to succumb to the gravitational pull, bringing it back to the equilibrium center (TPC., n.d.).

Concerns about digital technology use are often stated. While there are certainly concerns, it is important to grasp how far this "train" is out of the "station". Meaning, the concerns and issues which already exist, and will arrive in the future, are now about what do we do with what is already here; already integrated into our lives? How do we inform and manage the pendulum swing in ways that benefit rather than destruct? Helen Papagiannis poses in her book, *Augmented Human*, a hope for humankind. Her book is focused on the use of augmented reality (AR), however, I would stretch this to include all digital tools. She offers the following for consideration:

> *My wish for AR's legacy is that it elevates the experience of wonder and extends our imagination in new ways to inspire positive change in the world and humanity at large. One way AR can do this is as a powerful visualization medium. Seeing realities that are not yet actualized can stir our willingness to welcome and celebrate new possibilities, in turn expanding our consciousness to better humanity and activate change to benefit many. Let's make it our collective goal and commitment to design for the best of technology and the best of humanity. (2017, p. 132)*

References

Papagiannis, H. (2017). *Augmented human: How technology is shaping the new reality*. O'Reilly.

Stone, J. (2019). *Digital play therapy: A clinician's guide to comfort and competence*. Routledge.

Stone, J. (2022). *Digital play therapy: A clinician's guide to comfort and competence*, 2nd ed. Routledge.

TPC (n.d.). Pendulum motion. *The physics classroom*. https://www.physics classroom.com/class/waves/Lesson-0/Pendulum-Motion

7 Hardware and Software

There is certainly a wide variety of knowledge of and experience with both hardware and software within the psychological community. Technological advancements tend to move quickly, however, there are some basics that can be helpful to review. Whether you are quite savvy and already have quite an arsenal of hardware to use for different needs, or you are pretty new to all of it, conceptualizing hardware and software for clinical use can alter the approach in some ways.

Hardware

Professional and Personal

Having therapeutic digital tools can be exciting for the clinician and even their family members. A new iPad or virtual reality headset would look pretty exciting to use for personal reasons when not in the hands of clients. However, it is important to explore a few considerations before using professional hardware (and software) for both professional and personal purposes.

It is "cleaner" for multiple reasons to have equipment designated solely for your office. Clean in terms of work material stays at work, home material stays at home – the boundaries are clear and clean. Although it can be enticing to purchase a device with the intention of it serving both professional and personal needs, the chance for cross-contamination of information becomes exponentially higher if they are not kept separately. Purchasing one device for both can be a short-term gain but a long-term problem. Keeping your personal and professional equipment and data separate is important for ethical and tax-deduction purposes. If you have photos, videos, gaming accounts, or other items on the device, they can be accessed by the person using them (unless certain programs are password protected). The photos

DOI: 10.4324/9781003171799-7

you took of your last vacation with that device are now accessible for your clients, as well as that selfie your client took when you were not looking is now accessible by your family member. Even the most diligent clinician can become overwhelmed and forget to transfer information off the device. A device specifically designated for the office reduces such events. Additionally, separating the devices with personal and professional boundaries allows for the ease of being stored, charged, and secured in your office space.

The Home Office

As we learned quickly during the COVID-19 pandemic, the boundaries between home and office become a bit more blurred when working from a home office. A clinician's children may beg to play "just one game!" on the device. It is certainly tempting, however, just as one creates a private space in a home for home office telemental health use, it is important to keep devices separate and secured. Keep your work devices for work and your home devices for home. There are pros and cons to this as you may need to buy multiple devices. It can certainly be tempting for others in the home to use the devices, however, these boundaries serve multiple purposes.

Separation of Home and Work – Hardware

Keeping these boundaries clear can assist with yearly taxes and deductions, ethical concerns, and reduce accidental damage. A device used for both personal and professional use can result in confusion regarding the accurate percentage of time the device is used for personal versus professional purposes. As mentioned earlier, a device might have particular software or pictures relating to a client that would not be appropriate for anyone else to have access to. Personal use also increases the wear and tear and possibility of breakage, damage, or loss. Any of these scenarios could result in the device not being available for future sessions.

Specific Hardware Types

The advancements in hardware types will continue to excite and entice us over the years.

While clinicians do not need to be at the forefront, it will be important to pay some attention to what is being used both in the mainstream and also on the forefront. The digitally savvy clinician can continuously evaluate hardware and software for potential therapeutic inclusion. Here we will review the primary categories available early in the 21st century.

Digital Cameras

Prior to the inclusion of high-quality cameras on mobile smartphones, people often relied on traditional manual cameras with film or digital cameras. When evaluating any form of camera for therapeutic use, it is important to consider a number of factors. These can include the following: (1) for what will the camera/photographs be used? (2) how will the pictures be transferred into the client's health records? (3) which convenience features are important? (4) Will any photo editing be needed or desired? The answers will inform and guide the digital camera decisions.

As discussed earlier in the chapter, it is best to have a digital camera, in any form, designated for office use only. Evaluating the therapeutic purpose and the logistical process of inclusion in the session and the chart allows the clinician to make an informed purchase. A clinician who wants to edit photographs, for instance, would save time by using a smartphone or tablet to take the photos and an app on the device to edit the photos. Therapeutic practice management software on these devices allows for seamless transfer of the photos into the electronic health records or to collateral contacts. Connection via a charging cable or internet connection, i.e., Apple's AirPlay, also allows for transfers with logistical ease. Photographs may include artwork, sand therapy creations, and more. Proper permissions from the client/client's guardian and compliance with any governing boards will be critical to obtain prior to taking and transmitting photographs within session.

A manual camera requires rolls of film and processing of the film. This is time consuming, expensive, and difficult to include in a client's chart without a number of additional steps. Often the tasks that require additional steps are put aside to do "another time" and become a burden. Creating a process that is smooth and reliable allows the clinician to focus more on the therapeutic process and goals than the logistics of practice management. Therefore, a manual camera is not a viable option for many clinical settings.

A digital camera can be in the form of a stand-alone camera, smartphone, and/or tablet at this time. The benefit of the stand-alone camera is that it is separate from other content and uses. A smartphone or tablet may have other purposes and become complicated to leave in the office as a designated tool. One solution can be to use an older smartphone in lieu of the clinician's current phone. An older phone can be connected to the Wi-Fi for transfer of photographs without having carrier service or even via a charge cable (older ports may require an adapter to connect to a newer computer, but these can typically be found easily). This can be an economical way to designate a device for clinical use only.

Photographs are a fantastic way to preserve a client's work, particularly for child clients. The convenience of being quick, portable, downloadable, and printable allows the clinician to document the client's work without disrupting the flow of the session. The more fluid the routine system for transferring the photographs from the digital device to the electronic health records, the more reliable and less disruptive the process. A streamlined process for transferring the photographs allows the clinician to stay on task, remember whose work was being documented and when, and avoid misattributing a person's work unintentionally.

Smartphones

In addition to the camera function, smartphones can be used for a number of purposes in mental health treatment. A smartphone which is designated for the office only can avoid the cross-contamination of personal and professional information. This does not only apply to content such as personal apps, banking, and program notifications, but also personal text messages, email alerts, and more. Many notifications come through as banners across the top of the phone. This can be turned off and/or silenced in the settings menu of the phone, however, it can be completely avoided altogether if the phone is not used for personal reasons. If a phone has multiple uses, at best a deal for your local fast food restaurant comes across the screen; at worst another client call or text message comes across the screen. While it is best practice to not have your client's full name programmed into your phone, the content of the message or a unique first name, etc., could create a problem with confidentiality. It is best to avoid these dilemmas altogether with an office only device.

Searching for information through internet searches, watching videos, communicating, running thousands of different applications, and more can be an important part of the therapeutic interaction. These methods allow the client to convey information, emotions, and experiences, as well as share culture, interests, and more. Ethical considerations should always include protecting personal health information and confidentiality, and informed consent should be discussed and obtained in all situations.

Whether they are used during in-person or telemental health sessions, smartphones can be useful to access apps, web-based programs, as well as the camera function and access to a practice management software program. Smartphones have a convenient small size which allows for easy storage and access. The phone can be used with Wi-Fi enabled for access to the internet and/or transfer of information to specific designations. The clinician can also turn the Wi-Fi off as desired to further control how the phone is used in session (Stone, 2022).

Tablets

In 1987 the "Linus Write-Top" became an early version of a tablet. With a green screen and a stylus, the user could write on the screen and the computer would recognize what was written. The Write-Top was followed by the GridPad in 1989 by Palm, and in 1993 the early personal digital assistant (PDA), the Newton MessagePad, was launched by Apple. The PalmPilot PDA followed shortly thereafter with great success (Bort, 2013; Stone, 2022).

A prototype of the style of tablet we use today was launched in the year 2000 by Bill Gates. Apple revealed the first iPad in 2010 after a number of other tablet products were released. Over time many other products have been released with both hardware and software improvements. Understanding the breadth and depth of the features available will allow for the exploration of whether or not the new technologies are suitable for clinical use (Stone, 2022).

Tablets are being used in many different disciplines at this time for day-to-day business functions; within the service industry, schools, research, hospitals, and schools. They offer portability and power for many uses, including running apps, teaching, watching videos, presenting, collecting information and payments, sharing data, and more. Additionally, the touchscreen offers a kinesthetic experience as in interaction is generated with the hands (when not using a stylus) and this differs from the computer-person-mouse(touchpad) triad of a non-touchscreen device.

Surface area is another consideration when choosing clinical hardware. The smartphone screen is significantly smaller than many tablets and offer many of the same features. Stylus pens, additional cameras, and detachable keyboards are available as accessories for tablets to increase their function. Paired with Wi-Fi, the tablet can offer the functionality of the smartphone, with some of the features and abilities of a computer to improve the accessibility to a variety of programs and resources.

Gaming Consoles

The Maganvox Odyssey started the home gaming console craze in 1972. A boom followed in 1979 and continued into the 1980s and the Atari systems were launched. Sony, Sega, and PlayStation followed suit. Millions of people in US homes use in-home gaming consoles and companies such as Xbox, PlayStation, and Nintendo continue to develop their hardware and software (Njiri, 2016; Stone, 2022).

A gaming console is a unit which connects to a television screen or monitor. Handheld controllers translate the desired gameplay movements from the user to the program while being projected onto the screen. Controllers can be wireless (powered by rechargeable batteries) or wired (connected to the console by a cord). Controllers typically use buttons such as "X", "Y", "A", and "B" to make a character move around, jump, battle, and so forth, and also allows for selection of a variety of features (Stone, 2022).

A consideration regarding gaming consoles is the amount of space required for the storage and designated play area. The table or monitor stand, the monitor or television, any accessories, and seating can monopolize a fair amount of space in a clinician's office. When working in an in-person session, utilizing this amount of space can be a consideration. When working virtually, the space can be less concerning. However, if you already have a large monitor or television in your office, a traditional gaming console might be a great option to include in your digital therapeutics. These consoles offer an enormous library of games (software) which allows for both the clinician to choose/introduce games into the therapeutic setting and the client to suggest games to experience together.

Handheld Consoles

The 1970s quietly produced a number of digital technology advancements. The first handheld console launched in 1979 by Microvision. Early iterations were limited due to technical problems and a very limited supply of games. 1989 brought the first Game Boy, along with new features and software. Nintendo later developed the DS (Dual Screen) and PlayStation launched the PSP (PlayStation Portable) units (Codex Gamicus, 2019).

The Nintendo Switch has proven itself to have great value in therapeutic settings, particularly with children, adolescents, and young adults. Currently, there are two versions of the Nintendo Switch: the Nintendo Switch and the Nintendo Switch Lite. The benefit of the

Switch is that it includes two joycon controllers which can be removed and used by one or more people. Additional joycons can also be paired to include more than two players. Conversely, the Switch Lite has fixed joycons, as in, they cannot be removed and held independently of the unit or the other players. In-person sessions benefit from using the Switch as it can be preferable to have removable joycons so the client and clinician can each have one controller. A single player game becomes a two-player game when each person has a controller. Multiplayer games can be played by either pairing additional joycons so each person has two, or using multiple units to play simultaneously and join via the online connection. An accessory to consider is the Nintendo Dock. This allows the user to connect the unit to a larger monitor or television screen for easier viewing of the game play.

The Lite is most useful when using the Switch in telemental health sessions. In this scenario, the joycons are not being shared. It is important to note that users cannot connect in a multiplayer game unless the Nintendo online access has been purchased in addition to your Wi-Fi connection. If you will be using any form of multiplayer play with the Nintendo handheld consoles, both the online access and Wi-Fi connection will be necessary.

Computers

Borne from a need for efficiency in 1801, punch cards were invented by Joseph Marie Jaquard to automatically weave designs into fabric using a loom. The US census used this punch card technology in 1888 to assist with processing data – a reduction in the length of time to complete the census from 7 years to 3. The technological advancements between Jaquard's punch cards and now have been astonishing. The computers of the early 21st century culminate advances from the fields of math and science to provide us with many abilities we take for granted today. Interestingly, the first computer chip was created in 1958, the first mouse in 1964, and computers which once filled an entire room now fit into a small pocket (Zimmerman, 2017).

Computers can serve a number of purposes in a mental health clinician's office. A clinician may use a computer for their own clinical uses, case notes, research, and more. However, a computer can also be used for psychological testing, in-session research, resources, and/or in-session digital play. There are many types of computers available, so considerations regarding the choice of computer are similar to those for other types of hardware. These include: intended purpose, type of processor the intended software will need, memory, size, portability, psychometric testing use, and more (Stone, 2022). What you will use it for, with whom, in what way, and how many programs will you download/files will you save are all components which will contribute to the longevity of your computer in your office.

If there is a space concern and/or portability is important, then a laptop is a great choice. Laptops are certainly more portable and smaller than a desktop by design. Laptops can be equipped with powerful internal components which rival most desktops. For instance, if you would like a larger, separate monitor to view content on a larger screen, an external monitor can be connected. Being able to expand a laptop's functions increases the viability of this as a tool for the therapy office.

Although cost is clearly important, considering the purpose of the device may inform the decision making process. A less expensive device may need to be replaced more quickly due to lack of memory, poor graphics, and/or slow processing speed. Understanding what each of these parts contribute to the user's experience, along with the questions listed earlier, will help make the most of your investment and reduce frustration during use.

Extended Reality: Virtual Reality, Augmented Reality, and Mixed Reality

One of this author's favorite rabbit-hole-search finds is the discovery of the 1935 book, *Pygmalion's Spectacles.* Stanley G. Weinbaum penned this science fiction story in which the main character experiences "a fictional world through holographics, smell, taste, and touch" through a pair of goggles (p. 5). Less than a century later, these imagining by Weinbaum would be realized through virtual reality (Stone, 2022).

Guiding a client through the process of "try to imagine" or "let's paint a picture in your mind" certainly allows the exploration of topics, approaches, coping skills, catharsis, and more (Stone, 2022). The client can imagine a scenario in their mind. However, to communicate the scenario, the client must translate the mental images into words, verbally share the imagined situation or depiction, and hope that the description has conveyed a sufficient understanding of what was envisioned. The clinician must receive the auditory information, translate the words into images, and work to both visualize the scene and apply that to the therapeutic process. This is a very complicated interaction with numerous possibilities for misinterpretation. At times, the client draws or creates what is being imagined. This can help to minimize misinterpretations, however, there can be limitations in drawing abilities, limited mediums provided (i.e., pencils, crayons, markers, etc.), and the translation to the paper or other material is not always a true depiction of what was envisioned. A literal depiction can be less important at times, but for others it could make a significant therapeutic difference. With a customizable, immersive environment, the requested imaginings can be "created, entered, shared, experienced, and engaged with while both the client and clinician can bear visual and emotional witness" (Stone, 2022, p. 127). This is but one example.

Virtual Reality (VR)

Susanne K. Langer inspired Jaron Lanier when he coined the phrase "Virtual Reality", or VR, around 1985 (Virtual Reality Society, n.d.; Langer, 1955). A few of the components of VR that are particularly relevant and beneficial for use within the field of mental health include the experience of immersion, embodiment, and telepresence. The 360-degree vision field includes real-world content, computer-generated content, or a combination of both (Irvine, 2017). Mental health virtual reality (MHVR) synthesizes many of the desired elements and reduces the separation between the user and the machine. This interaction between user and machine more direct than we have ever had before (Bricken & Byrne, 1993). Tracking hand, head, and body movements in natural ways through the use of sensors contributes to a sense of congruency and immersion (Maples-Keller et al., 2017; Stone, 2022).

Multiple senses are engaged during the use of MHVR. The user's sight is restricted to the presented environment and stimuli. The sounds emanate from the headset. The autonomic sympathetic system can be activated, i.e., through fear inducing scenarios such as standing high on a cliff. The heart rate will increase, the sinking-stomach feeling can occur, and the lower brain regions discussed in Chapter 4 will prepare for a response. When using a VR headset, the user's mind and body believe they are in that environment. They embody their character/avatar, they interact with the environment and other characters. The user believes the scenario is real due to the immersive features of the programs. This is an important place where our concepts from chapter 3 integrate into the use of digital tools in therapy; one's sense of self, other, presence, interoception, theory of mind, perception, reality, self-awareness, consciousness, introspection, pretence, play, identification, representation, relationship, connection, and community.

Augmented Reality (AR)

Virtual reality is viewed through a headset which encompasses the eyes and allows the client to feel as though they are truly in that environment. Conversely, augmented reality (AR) is typically viewed through the camera feature of a smart device or specialized glasses. It includes computer-generated content which is shown as an overlay of the physical world environment (Stone, 2022). This content does not interact with the environment, instead it appears as a layer depicted over the real-world material; an overlay. An example could be of a computer-generated rabbit viewed through a phone's camera feature as a layer on top of the real-world environment. It may have animation, it may include sound, but it cannot interact with the environment, i.e., hop onto an existing chair. AR does not scan and input the environmental components for interaction. AR can also be used to translate languages (Irvine, 2017). The user launches the app in a smart device, holds the camera to the words in one language, and the app translates the words into a desired language.

Mixed Reality (MR)

Mixed reality extends the abilities of AR to include the ability for occlusion, or the ability for the computer-generated objects to interact with the environment (Irvine, 2017; Stone, 2022). If the rabbit were in a MR program, it would be able to jump onto the chair, behind it, and/or under it. With MR and occlusion, the computer-generated material interacts with the physical real-world environment to a greater degree. Irvine offers the following: "The general distinction is: all MR is AR, but not all AR is MR. AR is a composite. MR is interactive" (Irvine, 2017, p. 12). Dudley (2018) predicts that AR and MR might be/become more useful to users as they can be viewed through a smart device or glasses. The user does not need to be "sealed off in self-contained artificial environments" (Dudley, 2018, p. 6). However, this author would argue that for mental health treatment purposes, it could be the "sealed off" environment that allows for the therapeutic immersive experience (Stone, 2022). AR and MR have a place in therapeutic digital tool use, and these applications will surely become more relevant over time. The point is more that these are the considerations we must explore when utilizing these tools in an therapeutic setting.

What Hardware Is Needed For Clinical Sessions?

The hardware required to incorporate digital tools into mental health treatment can vary greatly. It depends on a few key considerations:

1 What types of software do you want to incorporate into your treatment? What will hold the most value for your client population?
2 Which of the identified software is cross-platform (works on multiple devices) and which types of hardware does it/do they run on?
3 How much room do you have in the therapy space/storage to keep the hardware? Do you want the devices to be stored in view or out of view of your clients?
4 What hardware devices do your clients have? Particularly useful when meeting via telemental health.
5 Do you work with multiple age groups and does this impact your decisions?
6 When making decisions about quality, try to consider the amount of use the device will withstand, the features included in conjunction with the features needed for therapeutic impact, etc. At times it might be appropriate to purchase "starter" devices with the knowledge they will most likely need to be replaced at some point, and other times it is better to buy the higher quality item initially.
7 Consider any accessories that will protect the device, prolong the life, assist with storage, etc.
8 Include both long and short-term goals. Hardware does not have to be purchased all at once.
9 Research models, features, reviews, prices (watch for sales), and ask trusted sources.
10 Consider any accessibility needs for your clients and consider any adaptation equipment available.
11 Consider whether or not you are able to provide loaner hardware for clients to use at home, i.e., during telehealth. (Stone, 2022)

The clinical purpose of the device should drive and inform the choice and the exploration of new releases will create a powerful repertoire of available clinical interventions.

Hardware Conclusion

Software will only run as smoothly as the hardware specifications allow (and original programming and coding of course). Ensuring you have fundamental knowledge in these areas will enhance the inclusion of the digital tools into your in-person and telemental therapeutic sessions. The chosen device(s) will provide a variety of experiences for the client, the clinician, and the client-clinician dyad. Periodic monitoring of upcoming hardware will allow the clinician to evaluate the components and possibilities for future inclusion in the mental health related work.

Troubleshooting Issues

Most people can identify simple troubleshooting concerns with their digital devices at this time. For instance, a low battery level or lack of available memory in the device can be relatively simple to spot. In other situations, issues can be the result of a necessary software update, issues with the device itself, or "bugs" in the software. The interactions between the hardware and software play off each other and are not mutually exclusive, so it is important to consider both when troubleshooting. The interplay between the software and hardware can impact your experience of the program you want to use. A simple way to troubleshoot is to search the internet for the name/model of your device + the issue you are having. Others have most likely had a similar issue and you might find a quick remedy pretty easily.

Battery Level

A device's battery level is important in many settings, however, it is quite important in a clinical setting. Being prepared for your session will include creating a system within which devices are charged regularly to ensure they are ready for use during a session. However, you do not want to keep your hardware plugged in or on a charge pad all the time. Not only is it a waste of energy, but older devices can be damaged by the constant influx of power. Newer devices can typically tolerate the constant power, but may overheat causing other damage (Hunt, 2022). Everything needs a break, including your devices.

Lack of Memory

Memory in a digital device is similar to working memory as discussed in neurology, education, and psychometrics. In hardware, working memory is discussed in terms of RAM. Nerds on Call state:

The memory is known as RAM. It is a part of your computer that it uses while it's powered on. Your computer stores everything that it's thinking about in RAM. If you're running a program, it's in RAM. If you're looking at a webpage, it's in RAM. RAM contains everything that's currently going on with your computer. And when RAM is in a computer that isn't powered, the RAM is empty. It's just waiting for something to think about. The more memory your computer has, the more it's able to think about at the same time. More RAM allows you to use more complex programs and more of them.

(Callnerds, 2019, para. 2)

For most hardware, the memory capacity is a fixed amount. If your device is sluggish, it could be a lack of RAM and it might not be eligible for an upgrade. Newer hardware often includes more RAM as our needs, uses, and expectations have increased over time. A first-generation iPad might have had 256 MB of ram, however, the newer models include 2 GB or more, depending on the model. The more detailed and/or feature heavy a program is, the more processing power and memory will be needed to run the program properly.

Lack of Available Memory

A lack of available memory can slow your device down or even cause if to turn itself off or shut down a program. At times, a program is unable to open due to a lack of available memory. It can be very helpful to close any unused programs. If that does not solve the issue, rebooting your device (turn it off completely, wait a minute or two, and then turn it back on, can help the device to reset, empty the trash, and be ready for the next task. At times items will need to be deleted to make more space on the device.

Storage

The device's storage can be likened to a closet; at some point it cannot hold more. Nerds on Call can help us understand storage further:

Storage refers to long-term storage. Everything that your computer knows, but isn't thinking about, is in storage, written on the Hard Disk Drive (HDD). This is a permanent type of storage: hard drives can be unplugged and contain the same information as when they're plugged in or turned on. Nothing actually gets changed on the hard drive: it gets pulled off the hard drive, into RAM/Memory. While it's in memory, you as the user can change it. When you save the information, it gets sent back to the hard drive storage in a different version. More hard drive storage allows you to store more things on your computer. However, it rarely affects your computer's performance. A computer with 1 gigabyte of RAM will work at the same speed whether it has 2 gigabytes of storage or 2000 gigabytes.

(Callnerds, 2019, para. 4)

Processor

The processor is the brain of the computer and referred to as the CPU or "chip". The CPU

takes instructions from a program or application and performs a calculation. This process can be broken down into three key stages: Fetch, decode, and execute. A CPU fetches the instruction from a system's RAM, then it decodes what the instruction actually is, before it is executed by the relevant parts of the CPU.

(Martindale, 2020, para. 6)

When troubleshooting for issues, consider that older devices with less RAM and a less-powerful CPU will have difficulties running newer, more content heavy programs.

Graphics

Many devices, such as tablets, phones, and consoles, have predetermined graphics (or video) cards included, without any choice given to the consumer. Computers have internal slots where a graphics card can be inserted or upgraded. If the graphics card cannot render (produce) the visuals required by the software, the result will be less than optimal visually. Visual stimuli can impact the engagement of the user, the level of immersion, and the overall motivation to use the digital tool/intervention.

Programming/Development Bugs and Glitches

Programming and development is more intricate than our needs, however a limited understanding of a few items could be helpful. Software is developed in different platforms, and these platforms have to be compatible with each other to create the proper user experience. When one platform makes a change, all the rest have to adjust to have the program work properly. There can be a time period between the first in line to make an adjustment, and the others working to adapt to the initial adjustment. This can create a "bug". Bugs can cause a feature that once worked well to now have an issue. The developer is most likely aware and will release an update or a "patch" to resolve the issue. Be sure to check for updates overtime, and certainly when you notice something is not working as it had previously, and you've already rebooted, checked for available memory, etc.

When information is not being properly processed by the CPU, "glitches" can happen. At times, something unexpected can happen and the aforementioned process can resolve it. One might never even know what really happened. Often a reboot of the hardware will solve the issue. If it does not resolve the issue(s), check for a software update. If the issue persists, there might be something larger happening within your device and a professional could be helpful. Before taking it in to someone, try the internet troubleshooting tip from earlier in this section, the model and make of the device + the issue, and see if you are able to manage it yourself.

If your program or app spontaneously quits, particularly in the middle of a session, it is important to not panic. If something is being created (art program, etc.), and can be saved, then it is recommended to periodically save regardless of any known issues. This can help to ensure the safe-keeping of any creation or even level of progress. Moderating your response to the temperament and needs of the client will yield the best result. Thankfully, most people are aware these things can happen and while it might frustrate, it is not an unknown phenomena, however, due diligence with your hardware and software can help to mitigate these issues.

Be Prepared

Being prepared will allow the clinician to work toward the 5Cs of using digital tools in a clinical setting. Having hardware charged, understanding enough about storage, processors, graphics, and memory, and some quick fixes when issues arise can continue a smooth therapeutic process. Becoming familiar enough so that you do not panic as the clinician will serve the client well when using digital devices.

Software

To differentiate from the term hardware, which includes the physical devices (phone, tablet, head mounted display unit, computer, etc.), software includes any programs, apps, procedures, and instruction associated with the operation of a particular computer system. Software includes a "set of instructions that directs a computer's hardware to perform a task is called a program, or software program" (Britannica, n.d., para. 1). This includes programs which "allow a computer to do a multitude of things" (typesof, n.d., para. 1). The software is mandatory for the hardware to execute complex functions for the user (Stone, 2022). System software, programming software, and application software are the primary types of interfaces between the software and the hardware. Understanding a few fundamentals can assist the user with troubleshooting a number of issues and help when communicating with a repair person.

System Software

System software orchestrates what the different parts of the system will do. This particular software is necessary to control the hardware's internal functioning through an operating system. This platform to run application software, along with internal checks and balances, gives the digital tool the ability to provide the desired user experience (ftms, n.d.). Also known as the operating system, the system software directs the hardware to execute a variety of commands (Britannica, n.d.).

A basic input/output system, also known as BIOS, starts the system when you turn on the device. This serves as a communication stream between the hardware and the operating system. There is also access between this system and the primary memory or RAM (random access memory). Internal ways to "clean up" and/or repair the system are also included (ftms, n.d.).

Utility programs and drivers (internal instruction manuals for the hardware device) are included in the operational software. Operational software "controls and manages the hardware and other software" on your device (Fisher, 2019, para. 1) and "manages and allocates memory space" (Amuno, 2019, para. 9). This type of software is typically specific to a manufacturer and/or a specific device. Examples include: Windows, Linux, Android, and Mac OS (operating system).

Programming Software

Programming software is primarily used by developers to create, debug, maintain, or support software programs and applications. If you hear the terms "compiler, debugger, text editor, interpreter, or linker", you are most likely listening to something referring to programming software. Some common programming languages include: C, C++, C#, BASIC, JAVA, Visual Basic, Phython, HTML, and PHP (ftms, n.d.). Different languages are used for different programming purposes and very few programmers know all of them.

Application Software

This is the software most non-tech savvy people are familiar with. Application software is designed for the end user or person wanting to use the device. This is the game, program, application (app), etc. we want to use; the one we purchase, download, and/or access. This type of software is not concerned with the functioning of the device, rather, it exists for whatever purpose the user has for accessing the device, i.e., create a document, play a game, access bank records, etc. Application software includes programs such as: spreadsheets, presentations, word processing, web browsing, graphic creation, games, and more.

When a user purchases a license to access a program, a license generator provides the license key and allows the person to have use the program. This process can be known to the user (a string of numbers/letters provided to input directly into the program) or internally without the user knowing the steps. Typically a user will agree to the conditions of the license use and pay the required fee prior to gaining access, unless a trial period is offered. A license allows the purchaser to access the software and each user would need their own license, depending on the end-user agreement. For instance, a company with 20 employees who all needed access to Microsoft Word would need to purchase 20 licenses to provide access to all the employees per the end-user agreement.

This text provides information regarding a few important systems. As with any digital technology, this information will be ever-changing. Key considerations include exploration of the available hardware and software as it is released, which hardware you choose to acquire, your knowledge of utilizing digital tools in therapeutic settings, and the needs of your clients.

Genres

Many people have attempted to classify the genres of software and there is not a clear consensus. However, Ha Lee et al. incorporated genres discussed up to 2014 and revealed the following:

1 Action: heavy emphasis on a series of actions performed by the player in order to meet a certain set of objectives
2 Action/Adventure: set in a world for the player to explore and complete a certain set of objectives through a series of actions
3 Driving/Racing: driving various types of vehicles as the main action, sometimes with an objective of winning a race against an opponent
4 Fighting: the player controls a game character to engage in a combat against an opponent
5 Puzzle: an objective of figuring out the solution by solving enigmas, navigating, and manipulating and reconfiguring objects modified from Wolf, 2001)
6 RPG: an emphasis on the player's character development and narrative components
7 Shooter: shooting at, and often destroying, a series of opponents or objects (Wolf, 2001)
8 Simulation: recreating an experience of a real-world activity in the game world
9 Sports: a simulation of particular sports in the game world
10 Strategy: players' strategic decisions and interventions to bring the desired outcome (modified from Apperley, 2006) (Ha Lee et al., 2014; Duckma, 2022).

There are a number of purposes for software as well. These can include: education, entertainment, exercise, meditation, party, social, fitness, food, travel, music, utilities, productivity, news, and dating (Ha Lee et al., 2014; Duckma, 2022).

A Guide for Choosing Software

The American Psychiatric Association created an "App Advisor" for assistance with choosing apps and other programs for clinical use. These questions can guide the clinician in the choice of programs for therapeutic inclusion. Please refer to Table 7.1 for this important guide.

In-Person and Telemental Health Session Considerations

Many digital tools have the flexibility to be used during in-person or telemental health sessions. However, compatibility between the hardware and software is important to investigate prior to the clinical use. If a clinician has a Hewlett-Packard Omnicept headset and the client

Table 7.1 Adapted from "App Advisor: An American Psychiatric Association Initiative", by the American Psychiatric Association, 2022, https://www.psychiatry.org/psychiatrists/practice/mental-health-apps/the-app-evaluation-model

Access and Background

1. Does the app identify ownership?
2. Does the app identify funding sources and conflicts of interest?
3. Does the app come from a trusted source?
4. Does is claim to be medical?
5. Are there additional or hidden costs?
6. Does the app work offline?
7. On which platforms/operating systems does it work?
   • Does it work on a desktop computer?
8. Does the app work with accessibility features of the iPhone/android?
   • Is it accessible for those with impaired vision or other disabilities?
9. Has the app been updated in the last 180 days?

Privacy and Security

1. Is there a transparent privacy policy that is clear and accessible before use?
2. Does the app declare data use and purpose?
3. Does the app describe use of PHI?
   • Deidentified vs. anonymous?
4. Can you opt out of data collection or delete data?
5. Are data maintained in the device or on the web?
6. Does the app explain security systems used?
7. Does the app collect, use, and/or transmit sensitive data? If yes, does it claim to do so securely?
8. What third parties does the app share data with?
9. If appropriate, is the app equipped to respond to potential harms or safety concerns?

Clinical Foundation

1. Does the app appear to do what it claims to do?
2. Is the app content correct, well-written, and relevant?
3. What are the relevant sources or references supporting the app use cases?
4. Is there evidence of specific benefit from academic institutions, publications, end-user feedback, or research studies?
5. Is there evidence of effectiveness/efficacy?
6. Was there an attempt to validate app usability and feasibility?
7. Does the app have a clinical/recovery foundation relevant to your intended use?

Usability (Subjective)

1. It offers minimal risk in terms of digital safety and privacy.
2. It appears to have some benefit.
3. What are the main engagement styles of the app?

(*Continued*)

Table 7.1 (Continued)

---

4. Do the app and its features align with your needs and priorities?
5. Is it customizable?
6. Does the app clearly define functional scope?
7. Does the app seem easy to use?

Data Integration Toward Therapeutic Goal

1. Do you own your data?
2. Can data be easily shared and interpreted in a way that's consistent with the stated purpose of the app?
3. Can the app share data with EMR and other data tools (apple Healthkit, FitBit)?
4. Is the app for individual use or to be used in collaboration with a provider?
5. If intended to be used with a provider, does the app have the ability to export or transfer data?
6. Does the app lead to any positive behavior change or skill acquisition?
7. Does the app improve therapeutic alliance between patient and provider?

---

has a Google Cardboard viewer (a phone is placed in a cardboard frame and three-dimensional materials are viewed), the two will not be compatible for a multiplayer experience. This is true for a number of hardware/software combinations. Asking the client what hardware and software they have available will assist the clinician to decipher what can be used in therapeutic sessions.

Clinicians will want to explore the following questions:

1   What will the therapeutic purpose of the digital tool serve within the client's treatment goals/plan?
2   What hardware and software does the client have access to?
3   Does the available hardware/software meet the known therapeutic needs?
4   If the answer to question number 3 is "no", then what hardware/software might meet the needs and what is the best way to gain access?

It is imperative that the clinical use of digital tools is most problem-free experience as it possibly can be to achieve the desired therapeutic goals (Stone, 2022). The due diligence of the clinician to identify the therapeutically appropriate hardware and software, combined with the clinician's theoretical foundation, informed consent, 5Cs (Competency, Culture, Comfort, Congruence, and Capability; Chapter 5), and experience will allow for the proper intervention assignment. Certainly inadvertent happenings will occur – a depleted battery, a low available memory, an app that needs updating – however, being knowledgeable about the hardware and software, creating a routine to ensure everything is up-to-date and in charged and working order, and routinely exploring new releases for future inclusion will ensure the best working environment for digital tool inclusion.

Conclusion

Carefully choosing software and understanding potential pitfalls will allow the play clinician to be well-prepared for the therapeutic inclusion of DPT materials. The mantra of "play it first, play it often, and play it more" applies to any and all of the software choices made. The new and exciting programs available will keep the client's motivation to engage high, and the multidimensional aspects will provide a tremendous amount of clinically relevant material whether your sessions are in-person or via telemental health.

References

American Psychiatric Association (2022). App advisor: An American Psychiatric Association initiative. *American Psychiatric Association.* https://www.psychiatry.org/psychiatrists/practice/mental-health-apps/the-app-evaluation-model

Amuno, A. (2019, February 8). Five types of system software. *Turbofuture.* https://turbofuture.com/computers/The-Five-Types-of-System-Software

Apperley, T.H. (2006). Genre and game studies: Toward a critical approach to video game genres. *Simulation & Gaming, 37*(1), 6–23.

Bort, J. (2013, June 2). The history of the tablet, an idea Steve Jobs stole and turned into a game-changer. *Business Insider.* www.businessinsider.com/history-of-the-tablet-2013-5

Bricken, M. & Byrne, C.M. (1993). Summer students in virtual reality: A pilot study on educational applications of virtual reality technology. In A. Wexelblat (Ed.), Virtual reality applications and explorations. Academic Press Professional.

Britannica (n.d.). Software. https://www.britannica.com/technology/software

Callnerds (2019). *What is the difference between memory and storage?* https://callnerds.com/whats-difference-memory-storage/

Codex Gamicus (2019, November 4). The history of handheld game consoles. *Fandom.* https://gamicus.gamepedia.com/History_of_handheld_game_consoles

Dudley, D. (2018, December). Virtual reality used to combat isolation and improve health. *AARP Magazine.* www.aarp.org/home-family/personal-technology/info-2018/vr-explained.html

Duckma (2022). What are the different types of mobile apps? *Duckma.* https://blog.duckma.com/en/types-of-mobile-apps/

Fisher, T. (2019, November 8). Types of software. *Lifewire.* www.lifewire.com/operating-systems-2625912

ftms (n.d.). *Computing basics.* https://ftms.edu.my/v2/wp-content/uploads/2019/02/csca0101_ch07.pdf

Ha Lee, J., Karlova, N., Clarke, R.I., Thronton, K., & Perti, A. (2014). Facet analysis of video game genres. *Ideals.* https://www.ideals.illinois.edu/bitstream/handle/2142/47323/057_ready.pdf

Hunt, C. (2022). Is it bad to leave your laptop plugged in all day while working from home? *Windows Central.* https://www.windowscentral.com/leave-laptop-plugged

Irvine, K. (2017). *XR: VR, AR, MR: What's the difference?* www.viget.com/articles/xr-vr-ar-mr-whats-the-difference/

Langer, S.K. (1955). *Feeling and form: A theory of art.* Scribner.

Maples-Keller, J.L., Bunnell, B.E., Kim, S.J., & Rothbaum, B.O. (2017). The use of virtual reality technology in the treatment of anxiety and other psychiatric disorders. *Harvard Review of Psychiatry*, *25*(3), 103–113.

Martindale, J. (2020, March 14). *What is a CPU?* https://sports.yahoo.com/cpu-210041849.html

Njiri, M. (2016, February 15). The history of gaming consoles. *Techinfographics.* https://techinfographics.com/the-history-of-gaming-consoles/

Stone, J. (2022). *Digital play therapy: A clinician's guide to comfort and competence*, 2nd ed. Routledge.

typesof (n.d.). *Types of software.* www.typesof.com/types-of-software/

Virtual Reality Society (n.d.). *The history of virtual reality.* www.vrs.org.uk/virtual-reality/history.html

Weinbaum, S.G. (1935). *Pygmalion's spectacles.* Project Gutenberg.

Wolf, M.J.P. (2001). *Genre and the video game.* University of Texas Press. https://www.academia.edu/435740/Genre_and_the_Video_Game

Zimmerman, K.A. (2017, September 7). History of computers: A brief timeline. *Livescience.* www.livescience.com/20718-computer-history.html

8   Case Examples

Reading about clinical cases can help to highlight the concepts within a text through practical examples. Through these examples clinicians may be able to connect aspects to their own clients or spark the imagination regarding other ways in which such tools could be therapeutically useful. These amalgamated cases have been chosen to illustrate a number of the concepts within this book. All case examples have been sanitized and altered in ways which diminish identification.

1   Sexual Trauma – Virtual Reality
2   Selective Mutism – Nintendo Switch
3   Anxiety, Relaxation – Virtual Reality
4   Accessibility, Differently-Abled – iPad Tablet
5   Self-Identity, Representation – Multiplatform

Sexual Trauma – Virtual Reality

Client: 30+ year-old woman

Hardware: HTC Vive Virtual Reality Head Mounted Display Unit (hmd)

Software: A boxing program*, followed by theBlu.
>   *the boxing program is not named as it has since changed from the time it was used with this client. There are a number of boxing games available and it is best to choose one based on the client's needs.

Janet, a woman in her mid-30s, experienced significant sexual trauma throughout her life. She presented for mental health sessions after a number of years of treatment with a few different therapists. Now a married mother of three, she recognized new difficulties which were

DOI: 10.4324/9781003171799-8

impacting her marriage and other relationships. She initially expressed concerns regarding emotional and physical intimacy; however, as treatment progressed it became more apparent that her sense of self, empowerment, responsibility, shame, fear, and more were impacting a number of aspects of her life.

Early sessions included gathering a thorough history and exploration of her concerns. She had a tumultuous relationship history with her primary caregiver. Her other caregiver was not present, which resulted in palpable grief and loss. The difficult dynamics of the primary caregiver relationship resulted in interpersonal relationship skills and expectations which fostered unhealthy early romantic relationships. It was within these relationships that Janet experienced sexual trauma, compounded by support systems which fostered the traumatic dynamic in the form of expectations of Janet to fulfill her "duty" as a partner, whatever was expected, regardless of her own needs or desires. The result was a myriad of emotional and psychosomatic symptoms, including muscle rigidity which caused significant pain.

Recognizing the importance of empowerment, appropriate responsibility, and catharsis, verbal accounts of events and emotions, along with timelines of events were created to further define and understand the components. The ripple-effect of the involved multidimensional dynamics emphasized the importance of further understanding. These understandings directly inform and impact the case conceptualization and treatment plan moving forward.

With primary goals of decreasing anxiety, increasing empowerment, and increasing a mind–body connection, virtual reality was introduced to Janet as a potential intervention. Virtual reality has been used for a number of anxiety, trauma, and exposure-based therapies. McMahon and Boeldt explored these concepts in their book, *Virtual Reality Therapy for Anxiety* (2022). Ioannou et al. (2020) performed a review of research regarding the use of virtual reality for the management of anxiety, depression, fatigue, and pain. Their analysis yielded support for the use of virtual reality with people experiencing these symptoms. Based on their review, they state: "VR intervention is more effective compared with the control (i.e., standard care) for anxiety, depression, fatigue, and pain" (p. 1).

Utilizing the Anxiety Cycle Model, MacMahon and Boeldt discuss the somatic, behavioral, cognitive, and genetic components of anxiety and then apply these to a variety of anxiety-based phobias and disorders. Key focal points include:

1   Anxiety management skills
2   Accessing fears
3   Experiencing relaxation and calm
4   Skill repetition and practice
5   Providing experiences which are positive and self-reinforcing
6   Preventing relapse (adapted from McMahon and Boeldt, 2022, p. 29)

Virtual reality can provide the user with the unique simultaneous experiences of other and current. The "other" is a multisensory environment other than the physical one the person is in. The "current" includes the person is in their physical environment, with at least one other person (therapist), and encompasses their own complex being. Janet was interested in an experience which allowed her to safely embody another personality to express and act on feelings she had difficulty claiming; namely, expressions of anger, rage, and violence. Each of these resided within her, but her family of origin expectations did not allow for acceptance or expression of them in any way.

Janet utilized a boxing game through Viveport, a subscription-based platform through which users can access thousands of virtual reality programs. She chose the game herself from those offered. After a brief orientation to the virtual reality head mounted display unit (hmd), the controllers, and features of the HTC Vive, she was ready to go! She practiced movements and actions through the tutorials to familiarize herself with the expectations of the program. She was able to choose her opponent and decided upon a male character who appeared less than honorable, somewhat of a stereotypical "pimp" type character. She bent her knees and held up her gloves, ready to face her opponent.

Even before the match began, it was apparent that Janet had received from the therapist and environment and also given herself permission to release emotions, actions, and reactions she had not been able to embody in the past. Her typical stance was timid and reserved, however, here stood this woman in a powerful and protective stance, ready to face what appeared to be a perpetrator of the negative sexual experiences of her life. The difference was remarkable and she had not even begun the active portion of the program.

When the opponent began to speak to her, "trash talk" if you will (casting doubt on her abilities to defend herself or be victorious), she began to respond with powerful retorts – such as: "you can't hurt me", "I am going to f* you up", and "you'll never do any of that to me again". She invited the character to "come at" her and start the fight.

When the bell rang she unleashed. She pummeled the character round after round and verbalized many emotions. It appeared as though years of pent-up emotions and experiences finally had an acceptable avenue of release. After a few rounds in the boxing ring, he had been defeated in more ways than one; in the ring, in her body, and in her mind.

Janet stood in the office, appearing taller and stronger, chest heaving from the activity, and sweat across her face. Through the visual stimuli, the auditory speech and cues, along with the lateral and bilateral movement, Janet was able to activate multiple brain regions, access her emotions, experiences, cognitions, and memories, and express them. With the hmd on, one could only see the lower part of her face clearly and it was unmistakable that she now donned a very large smile. Janet celebrated her victory against the perpetrator and the release of that which had never been acceptable. She stated, "I finally got to do that! I've been waiting so long". It was a phenomenal moment; witnessed by the therapist through a casted image on a screen and by watching her physical being in the room.

The boxing experience of that day was complete and her sympathetic nervous system was in full confrontation mode. To assist Janet with activating her parasympathetic system, we began by regulating her back to the physical environment (she kept the hmd on by her own choice). By speaking to her and gently touching her arm (with her verbal permission), she began to rejoin the room and interact more with the therapist. She spoke about the experience and how freeing it had been to act in ways she had never been able to before. She threw her arms up in a "Rocky Balboa"-type stance to signify her victory. She was strong and proud. Verbalizing her experience was important for her to move from full arousal toward a more relaxed and homeostatic, parasympathetic state.

It was suggested by the therapist that a more relaxing and regulating program be used prior to leaving the session. theBlu program was chosen as a calming, peaceful environment. theBlu has three portions, the first of which is an underwater scene with sea anemones, sea cucumbers, fish, coral, turtles, and jellyfish. The movement of the user and interaction with the environment is minimal. Initially she commented on the colors and populated portions of the environment. She chose to sit on the carpet and employ some deep breathing to relax from the high activity of the boxing. Her speech slowed and she was able to relax into the cadence of the ocean. She remarked how peaceful it was and she was visibly comfortable and relaxed. This was a markedly different posture than she had during the boxing.

The use of theBlu, or another parasympathetic-inducing program, allows a person to utilize anxiety management skills. Common skills include diaphragmatic breathing, progressive muscle relaxation, mindfulness, and imagery (McMahon & Boeldt, 2022). Utilizing these skills can reduce the state of nervous system arousal through body and mind awareness and connection. Janet was able to move from a "wild-eyed" limbic brain response state to a relaxed, present, connected state.

She removed the hmd and her gaze returned to the therapist. With an enormous smile she stated, "that was really incredible, I want to do that again next time!". Over time, through this activity and processing of the experiences, Janet was able to further distinguish between her family of origin's beliefs and expectations and her own. She was able to express her emotions and experiences through the highly cathartic process. Subsequently, further therapy sessions focused on pairing the experiences within virtual reality with experiences and dynamics in her day-to-day life, and she was able to define her boundaries and parameters for herself. Virtual reality was a very powerful tool for Janet to access and express thoughts, feelings, and emotions she was unable to previously, and then pair those experiences with important self-concepts which impacted her sense of herself in the world within her own desired definitions.

Selective Mutism – Nintendo Switch

Client: 6–8 year-old male

Hardware: Nintendo Switch

Software: Legends of Zelda, Breath of the Wild
*adapted from Stone, J. (2020a), *Digital Play Therapy*, 1st ed., pp. 219–223.

John was a third-grade student who presented for play therapy treatment for selective mutism with his mother. John's mother reported that he was experiencing a significant amount of anxiety regarding social communication, particularly at school, during afterschool activities, and with people he did not know. He would frequently shut down, turn away, and hide under furniture when he had to verbally interact with others. Thankfully, John attended a small school which accepted and accommodated his needs in this area; however, as he rises in grade and academic expectations, his level of anxiety was becoming more of a hinderance.

Initially John did not want to come to the play room alone (without his mother). During the first session, John sat very close to his mother with his arms intertwined with hers and avoided eye contact with the therapist. The first two sessions included John and his mother with a verbalized goal of titrating toward an individual session. Over time, he willingly participated in the activities and his anxiety appeared to decrease as he felt more safe and secure with the therapist in the environment and interactions. Once began sitting further away from his mother and his posture relaxed, suggestions for the mother to stay in the waiting room were met with little resistance. John began to attend sessions without his mother.

During the first session alone with the therapist, the gains John had made during the weeks before seemed to vanish. Instead of interacting, John sat uncomfortably in the corner on a *Hugibo*® pillow. The therapist reminded John of his options within the office, including that he was free to explore the room and choose what he would like to do. Based on the observations of his nonverbal behavior, it appeared that his anxiety was worsening as the session progressed. The therapist opted for a parallel play route and started to play with nearby magnet tiles. Through narrating the play, the therapist hoped that John would become interested. John's posture and stance did not change.

When it became evident that the magnetic tiles were not enticing John into collaborative or cooperative play, the therapist put the magnet tiles away. John had pointed to the Nintendo Switch previously and his mother had shared that he watched his older brothers play in the past. They frequently left him out of the play as he was the youngest of the siblings. The chosen game was *Zelda, Breath of the Wild*. John was quite excited. In order to play together with one Nintendo Switch, the therapist removed the joy con controllers from each side and placed the center screen on a flat surface; the screen was propped up and facing the direction where John was sitting. John began tracking the therapist's movements and it appeared he hoped he could play too. The therapist spoke about a few details of the game play. She began to play the game while narrating the process, some frustrations about a quest, and concerns about trolls in the area. The therapist wanted to have John join the play and once interest was apparent, she said to John directly, "usually kids in here use this left-hand controller and we play together. I am not very good at the left-hand controls so if you decide you want to help, I would be very grateful". As John inched closer and closer to the therapist. Once he was close enough and without making eye contact or verbalizing anything that acknowledge his involvement, the therapist passed over the left-hand controller.

Some readers might not be aware of the Nintendo Switch or Legends of Zelda, Breath of the Wild, so a brief description will be given here.

Nintendo Switch

The Nintendo Switch is a handheld gaming console which includes a center screen and two joy con controllers, one placed on each side of the screen. Accessories can enhance the use of the switch by pairing additional controllers and/or using a dock to project the images through a larger computer monitor or television screen.

A great benefit of the Nintendo Switch is that the controllers can be used independently from the main unit and from each other (not the Lite model). Each controller has different functions and abilities. As an example, the left controller has the ability to make the main character, Link, walk and change directions. However, if a person wants to look around or have a different viewpoint, the left controller cannot accomplish this. Therefore, if two different people each have one controller, they must work together to accomplish both simple and complex tasks. The communication between the two players is critical for the game play, including accomplishing goals and self-preservation (defending oneself, not falling off a cliff, etc.).

Legends of Zelda

The Legend of Zelda, Breath of the Wild game is an action-adventure game which was released in 2017 (Nintendo, 2017, para 1). Legend of Zelda is a franchise game with the original having been released in Japan in 1986. This game has developed in many directions since the 1980s (Fandom, n.d., a). The main protagonist, Link, is the eternal hero in each installment (Fandom, n.d., b, para 1). Link adventures through the countryside of Hyrule, exploring a variety of landscapes, defeating monsters, navigating challenges and quests, collecting items, and helping others. Breath of the Wild is considered an "open-world game" where players can explore Hyrule as they choose. The ultimate goal of the game is to defeat the evil character Ganon and the player can complete the game's tasks in any order they desire (Cooper, 2017, para 3). Ganon has been locked away in the Hyrule Castle with future evil plans and it is Link's task to save the land (Stone, 2020b).

John

Playing Legends of Zelda was a highly motivating activity for John. The hope was that it would be motivating enough for John and he would engage in the game play and with the therapist to coordinate movements and efforts toward particular goals. One scene involved walking through a field to get to another area of the map. The therapist decided to test the limits and did not automatically change the point of view to follow the path John had Zelda walking. This resulted in Zelda almost walking into danger. Suddenly John exclaimed verbally, "RUN OVER THERE!" He pointed to the left and stood up, a bit exasperated. The verbalization was a first between the two, however, it was not highlighted as an event. The game play continued.

Over the time John played Zelda in session, there were quite a few instances when John did not communicate his needs or desires within the game, verbally or nonverbally. The lack of communication led to a variety of events, including interactions with enemies and inadvertently entering dangerous territories. The main character of the game, Link, can encounter a variety of dangers during the game play, including skeleton-like creatures called stalkoblins, trolls called bokoblins, flying keese, and more. Our Link character was attacked multiple times by creatures and a lack of communication between the therapist and John left Link vulnerable. At times, Link fell off cliffs and once he missed out on catching and taming a horse. Now that John began to verbally communicate with the therapist, albeit sparce, the pair could briefly pause the game to allow time to regroup, discuss goals and tactics, and process any necessary changes. Environmental cues, such as music changes when danger was close by, were recognized and discussed, along with strategies when these cues happened, such as ways to alert the other person. These conversations allowed for better team cohesion, strategy, and plans for future communication. Once the game was un-paused, the play was able to continue with greater success.

Soon, John became increasingly aware of the benefits of communicating verbally with another person about what he wanted to result from an interaction. Over time John became quite verbal about what he thought should happen in the game at any given moment; sometimes the exuberance was unwarranted. This allowed the therapist and client to work on self-moderated communication skills. It became apparent that it was time to work on the next level skills of teamwork and communication once he was confidently coming into the play room, getting out the switch, and giving the right hand joy con controller to the therapist.

At times, the therapist would reflect what the experience was like when John would demand certain things, not work as a team, and not have space for the goals of both players. Based on the history provided by the mother initially, and a collateral contact conversation with his teacher, it appeared that a number of response patterns shown during the Zelda play were being enacted in other environments. A number of questions arose for the therapist: 1. Does John remain quiet in other environments until he is motivated to engage and then tries to take over and control the situation? 2. Once John tries to control the situation do his peers reject him? 3. How did John experience these rejections?

John's response patterns appeared to exacerbate and reinforce some of what John was already integrating about his perceived place in the world: he felt he was not acceptable when he was a silent, withdrawn person, however, he acceptable as an outspoken person either based on people's typical reaction to him when he was exuberant. John had difficulties with recognizes his own contribution to these dynamics. He also struggled with any moderation of his responses which could potentially result in more satisfactory outcomes. Future sessions included John and the therapist exploring these concepts further and generalizing the Zelda play to his day-to-day social experiences.

It became apparent that John had difficulties within uncomfortable situations. He struggled to moderate his responses in multiple environments, just as he had within the Zelda play. If John felt inferior in some way within an interaction, then he responded in a one of two ways: "all-in" with a need to control the situation or "all-out". When he was all-in, he could prevent himself from feeling too vulnerable. When he was all-out, he could feel (relatively) unaffected by the situation. Neither of these approaches felt sufficient to him nor did they meet his needs, as he had a strong desire to be accepted by others and included in activities.

After some time, John was requesting to play other games in sessions. He wanted to play other Switch games, as well as board games. The patterns identified in the last paragraph were applied to each type of game, withdraw or control. The therapist focused on a number of concepts within this game play, including a significant amount of mirroring, modeling, and processing. One goal was to assist John with an increased level of self-awareness. The hoe was that once he truly understood the patterns of his interactions and his responsibility in them, he could more intentionally choose to his responses. If he chose not to alter his responses, it would indicate that his need for something else was stronger than his need for the improved social interactions. Dependent upon the insights and discoveries during treatment, the treatment plan/goals were altered. As a fundamental concept, if you can identify the motivations and/or needs in a situation, and address it/them, the internal drive for change is exponentially increased.

The Zelda game play yielded some exciting information. As a review, John was able to engage well in play activities with the therapist first with his mother present and then again when his mother was not, after a readjustment period. The use of the Nintendo Switch became a highly motivating digital tool. Zelda, Breath of the Wild proved to be a game which offered particular play components that revealed and highlighted some of John's social difficulties. His response patterns were relatively consistent and appeared in his board game as well. This consistency gave strength to the clinical working hypotheses. During both digital and board game play, John was encouraged to tolerate the gray areas between the black and white polar ends. The sense of safety and trust in the therapeutic relationship allowed John to experiment with the gray areas. As an example, John worked on reciprocal interactions instead of attempting to gain full control of everything. Teamwork became a way to improve communication, not only in the logistics of it, but also the value it provided to the game play – which was much more motivating for John. Considering what the two players might want to accomplish as a team instead of individual, unspoken goals led to more positive results. The importance of also considering what each individual player might want separately arose, and therefore the exploration of how that could be supported by each player and then integrated into the general game play. For John, the more successes he experienced, the more motivation he had to continue; both within the session and in his day-to-day life. As is true with most humans, the more motivation he had, the more progress he made. Additionally, the more progress he made, the more confidence he had to continue these new skills outside of the play therapy room.

The activities and interventions employed during the sessions with Jack were very well suited for his needs and desires. Highly motivating activities increased his personal resilience and kept him moving forward in his self-awareness, growth, and response pattern changes.

John's mother shared successes he was experiencing due to his attempts to utilize different social responses and interactions during his interactions with peers. He was able to practice these skills during periodic activities (such as afterschool play), structured around an activity, and time limited. Remaining sessions were focused on his attempts to alter his social interactions and responses so he can generalize the successes to his school interactions. A follow-up call to John's teacher informed her of the work to date and allowed collaboration regarding continued support for John to experience ongoing success in school. After the conclusion of the therapeutic work, his mother emailed updates regarding John's greatly improved social interactions and his increasing participation in required and nonrequired group activities. The safety of the relationship, along with the inclusion of a highly motivating, complex digital tool and program, allowed for numerous opportunities to identify and intervene in patterns and behaviors that restricted John from what he considered (as opposed to defined by others) positive social interactions.

Anxiety, Relaxation – Virtual Reality

Client: 12–14 year-old female

Hardware: Phone, Oculus Quest 2 Virtual Reality Head Mounted Display Unit

Software: Meme searches, NatureTreks

Tori is an early adolescent female client who presented with symptoms of anxiety, depression, and interpersonal trauma. Family acrimony and discord, along with multiple moves, losses, and disruptions, have led her to strive toward compartmentalization and emotional avoidance. Her relationships with her parents had diminished and she was experiencing a high level of anhedonia. She was not internally motivated to attend therapy sessions and presented with a blank stare and numerous audible sighs.

Tori was quite slow-to-warm within the therapeutic relationship. Forced to attend by her parent, she resisted engaging with the therapist until a phone notification revealed meme interactions between her best friend and herself. She revealed that she and her friend rarely texted sentences or paragraphs to each other, rather, they sent memes to each other which conveyed a variety of messages, emotions, and experiences, etc. Interactions between the therapist and Tori began to center around finding particular memes and sending them to each other in session. This allowed for some distance between the two while interacting and sharing details about a variety of topics. Tori would sit on the floor against a large stuffed animal and the therapist would sit on a nearby futon couch. Eventually the sessions were full of laughter and connection as more memes were shared.

Initially the memes were lighthearted and silly; a cat in a precarious position or a baby making an unexpected facial expression. Over time, memes with a more serious meaning were shared, many which expressed a level of darkness, depression, and fear that Tori could not or would not put words to. These expressions allowed a window into her anxiety, fear, and depression. She was not hopeful for any improvement or change and had rare positive feelings, predominately when she was texting with her friend.

Once a more positive rapport had been established, the focus shifted to a desire to identify ways to regulate herself and feel safe. She reported that interactions with her sibling, and witnessing interactions between her parents and sibling, resulted in her feeling fearful and wanting to withdraw to her room. Her sibling and parents argued a lot and while there were no physical altercations, the verbal interactions were heated and loud. She spent a large amount of her time at home in her room, either reading books or texting on her phone.

Some of the activities highlighted in example number one, such as diaphragmatic breathing, progressive muscle relaxation, mindfulness, and imagery were discussed taught to provide both language and activities for Tori to utilize wherever she might be. Working toward identifying a safe space began with art materials and a variety of memes. Ultimately, though, much of what came to light in these sessions was limited by and inability to translate the components into day-to-day existence.

Therapeutic virtual reality was introduced to Tori as a possible way to really experience and identify a safe space (Stone, 2021a, 2021b). She was familiar with virtual reality as her sibling owned a Sony Play Station headset. There are some differences between her brother's hmd and the one in the therapist's office, but overall they are very similar, therefore the transition to use was quite smooth and required minimal acclimation.

The process to identify what safe felt and what that might look like for her was difficult until virtual reality was utilized. Trauma-informed virtual reality play therapy was employed (Stone, 2021a). Through a virtual reality program called NatureTreks, Tori was able to choose from a variety of environments. Each has the goal of providing a relaxing, meditative experience for the user. Tori entered a number of the worlds. She was able to look through as many as she wanted in an effort to identify an area within that she identified as allowing her to feel safe. Ultimately she chose the meadow environment. This area is very green and lush, with plants, trees, and flowers all over. There are animals such as rabbits and deer strolling by. Beyond choosing an environment, the goal was to identify a space within the environment that felt safe to her. Noting the details was important. Certain sights, sounds, and environmental cues were taken into consideration. After exploring the green meadow, she identified an area next to some large boulders as an area which felt safe.

Tori used the array of tools within the program to customize her area. An array of options allows the user to grab and/or throw orbs to place rocks, trees, flowers, and more as desired. Tori opted to place a number of rocks to encircle her. She also placed trees around the rocks for an additional layer of protection. Flowers, plants, trees, rocks, and butterflies surrounded her. She laid down on the floor and looked around the environment. From the casted two-dimensional view (the therapist was watching from a computer monitor screen), the therapist could see the view from the floor, looking up at the majestic boulders and trees surrounding her. It appeared as though no one could get in or out without her permission or knowledge. The therapist was able to watch Tori regulate right before their eyes; a lowered breathing rate, relaxed muscle tone in the face and body, and a decrease in verbal narration transformed this hypervigilant, dysregulated, anxious young teen into a calm, peaceful, regulated person who was enjoying the mindfulness of her environment.

Once she reached this peaceful state, she promptly fell asleep. In what might seem to be an odd statement, the fact that she fell asleep was an enormous accomplishment. Reminding ourselves of her initial presentation, she was full of eye-rolls, audible sighs, and minimal eye contact. She had not felt safe enough to engage with the therapist or the environment. Slowly she was able to engage through a third party, memes, and begin to feel a sense of physical and interpersonal safety. At this point she has progressed to occupying space in relatively close proximity to the therapist, laying down on the floor with a headset on, which is a vulnerable position, and falling asleep. It was astounding.

Tori was an extremely hypervigilant young person who created a space within NatureTreks, within which she felt safe enough to fall asleep. This really speaks to the power of the immersion of virtual reality and the program which provided an environment she could identify as feeling safe and the further customize to her needs. Her parasympathetic nervous system and default mode network could activate and allow her to relax and enjoy the space she had created.

After waking her, she and the therapist identified the components of the safe area. The colors, sensations, sounds, etc., all worked together to create this space for her. Once the components were identified they could be used to recreate this environment, and hopefully the experience, within her home. She began to brainstorm different ways she could use existing space and materials in her room to mirror this experience.

Tori had green tapestries and many pillows in her room. She decided to use a corner as the two walls were solid and sturdy like the large boulders. She hung the tapestry across the two walls and propped a beanbag and a variety of stuffed animals around in a rough circle. She hung a string of twinkle lights across the top to simulate the dark, start studded sky she chose in NatureTreks. She found music on Spotify that she identified as relaxing. This spot was used to escape the household stress and tension, to read, to chat with her friend, and to relax. Once she completed the space, she sent an array of photos to the therapist.

Amazingly, she moved mid-treatment and recreated the space in her new home. This safe space creation was done spontaneously – without the therapist prompting – indicating a high level of importance for the space in her life. Treatment was continued virtually and she was able to share her space with the therapist through a webcam. Trauma-informed virtual reality play therapy provided the environment, control, creativity, and connection she needed to feel safe and the therapist-client relationship allowed her to identify what it all meant to her.

Accessibility, Differently-Abled – iPad Tablet

Example A

> Client: 10-12 year-old female
>
> Hardware: iPad Pro tablet, 12.9"
>
> Software: Virtual Sandtray App, therapist version

Marie was a latency aged client who was experiencing difficulties related to family of origin disruption and an unknown degenerative motor disease. Adjusting to both situations was quite difficult as both had unknown future trajectories. The family of origin disruption included a rejection of Marie due to her physical limitations and needs. The degenerative disease was constantly being evaluated by specialist after specialist, with no medical diagnosis or treatment plan in sight. Both left Marie in a state of the unknown; disruption, instability, and anxiety with no known neuroception of safety on the horizon.

Over the course of treatment, Marie's ability to control her own limbs decreased rapidly. Initially she was able to walk into the office using crutches and access a majority of the tools available, but within a few months she was utilizing a motorized wheelchair to get around. At first she was able to easily use her limbs, but then over a relatively short time she could not predictably use her arms or legs. Prior to this change in mobility, a favorite activity of hers was to use the traditional sandtray.

Some readers might not be aware of sand therapies, so a brief history and description will be given here.

Sand Therapies

Sand therapies encompass a variety of interventions stemming from the work of Dr. Margaret Lowenfeld. Beginning in 1929, she started utilizing an intervention called the Lowenfeld World Technique. Prompted by the experiences of children during wartime, she sought a way to allow children to express themselves non-verbally through a "multidimensional language" (Lowenfeld, 1954). "I set for myself as a goal to work out an apparatus which would put into the child's hand a means of directly expressing his ideas and emotions, one which would allow of the recording of his creations and of abstracting them for study" (Lowenfeld, 2007, p. 3). The Lowenfeld World Technique consisted of the creation of a world which requires no specific skill or talent, and "facilitate expression of concepts and of inner experience which are outside the framework of even 'phantastic' drawing and modelling" (Lowenfeld, 1954, p. 1). Clients chose "world objects" or miniature items to place into the tray of sand to create a world.

Lowenfeld set the specifics for the World Technique which included a tray of metal or wood with a metal lining painted blue, world objects, sand, and water (Lowenfeld, 1954). The tray was to be placed on a table and be smaller than the table so items could be placed on the edges during construction of the world. Sand is placed in the tray and is of medium coarseness. She suggested one could have two trays with varying coarseness of the sand. She suggested one should have a complete set of objects, but not too grand a collection that would overwhelm the creator. The objects would have both conventional and symbolic value.

Dora Kalff traveled to train under Dr. Lowenfeld at the urging of Dr. Carl Jung. After training under Lowenfeld for a year, Kalff returned and created an offshoot of the World Technique (frequently referred to as Sandtray Therapy now). Kalff named her version

Sandspiel, or Sandplay. There are other sand therapies to date, but Sandtray and Sandplay are the two primary versions used in the 21st century. For more information, readers can seek out books writing by Homeyer & Sweeney (2016) and Homeyer & Lyles (2022).

Marie had enjoyed using the traditional sandtray prior to her increasing motor difficulties. Once she was using the motorized chair, it became difficult to move close enough to the table and tray to reach the sand or even to choose her own objects to place. As her limb movements became more spastic and uncontrollable, she became more distraught, frustrated, and saddened that her body would not cooperate any longer. It was difficult in-and-of-itself, but also because it was symbolic of the difficulties she was having in life overall: nothing was as she hoped or wanted and she had no control over herself or anything else.

Virtual Sandtray®©

Around the same time, this author co-created the Virtual Sandtray®©, a digital version of the Lowenfeld World Technique, or sandtray therapy. Created in response to the 2011 Tōhoku earthquake and tsunami in Japan, the Virtual Sandtray App, or VSA, was designed for use by people for whom and places in which the traditional sandtray setup was not possible. Grounded in Lowenfeld's principles, the VSA allowed Marie to create worlds in her lap using a 12.9" iPad tablet. When she began to create her first tray with the VSA she looked up to the therapist and exclaimed "I CAN DO THIS!" The therapist responded, "yes, you CAN!".

Providing a variety of interventions and tools for use in therapy speaks to the importance of cultural sensitivity, humility, and accessibility. Even if the needs are not as specific as Marie's, different tools and interventions will speak to people in different ways, at different times, and with different meanings, depending on the needs of the client at that time. One size does not fit all, and while clients might be able to improvise or compromise, there are times when the "right" medium allows the flow of expression in a way that an improvised/compromised one cannot.

Marie was able to create world depictions in the Virtual Sandtray App with relative ease. She commonly depicted family scenes, isolation, loneliness, frustration, anger, rejection, and aggression. She longed for what she considered a "normal" life with her parents and siblings, and a body that responded to her desired movements. Her ability to create and express emotions and experiences allowed her to release them, understand them, grieve for what she felt she had lost, and begin to assess what the future might hold. For her there were not a lot of answers, but having the tools to express herself within the container of a safe space with a trusted professional allowed her to move closer toward acceptance of her situation and support through the unknowns.

Example B

Client: 30+ female

Hardware: iPad Pro tablet, 12.9"

Software: Virtual Sandtray App, therapist version

Jennie was a graduate student in her early thirties. She presented to therapy to process some life decisions and directions. She lived alone and was at the point in her life where she desired a partner and family. Relationship struggles had led her to question whether or not she was capable or worthy of a long term, healthy relationship.

Her parents had been married for decades and she felt they had a solid relationship. Her brother had a wife and children, and she felt like she was the odd-person-out in the family. A student in psychology, Jennie attempted to apply her psychological knowledge and education to the therapeutic process, which led her to remain in her "academic/ intellectualized" brain and not allow her emotional experiences to enter into the therapeutic process. After a few failed attempts to elicit emotional reactions, another approach was introduced: the Virtual Sandtray App.

Presented as a tool for her to "check out", she was eager to give an opinion about this digital version of a sandtray. She began to experiment with the features and controls and when she felt comfortable, a world began to emerge. The only prompt given by the therapist was a request to try out this new tool.

Jennie began by digging down in the sand to the liquid layer (just as the Lowenfeld tray was painted blue on the bottom). This digging created a horizontal line of water across the tray, essentially diving the tray in half. On the upper portion of the tray, she placed a home, flowers, trees, two adult women, two children, and a dog. She painted the sand with grass and it depicted a very happy, family oriented scene. On the lower portion of the tray she placed dead, broken trees, a bleached cattle skeleton, and three adults – two women and a man – in a triangle shape, shoulder to shoulder, looking outward.

Essentially, they were all looking in other directions and not at each other. They were connected but disconnected. The lower half of the tray appeared desolate, lonely, void of color or happiness, and broken.

When Jennie completed the scene she handed the tablet to the therapist. She asked, "what do you think?". The therapist looked at the tray and handed the tablet back to Jennie, "what do YOU think?". She looked at the tray in a very pensive manner. Her eyebrows began to furl with concern. She looked back up to the therapist's gaze and said, "I think I need to come out to my parents".

In this case the projective, creative sandtray intervention allowed the brain to bypass the executive functioning process enough to have the emotional content of the amygdala and thalamus to come through. In her mid-thirties she had never publicly acknowledged her sexual preference which led to her abstaining from relationships and thereby depriving herself of a life she truly desired.

After processing the tray and her realizations, the therapeutic sessions centered on her identity, conversations she wanted to have with others in her life, relationships, and a life plan she had not allowed herself to contemplate previously. Thankfully her family's response was positive, and she continued to work on the above goals. Future work surrounded the navigation of new relationships.

Self-Identity, Representation – Multiplatform

Client: 10–12 year-old male

Hardware: Multiplatform: PC, Mac, iOS, Android, Amazon Devices, Xbox One, Oculus Rift, and HTC Vive. (Roblox, 2022)

Software: Roblox
*excerpts about Roblox adapted from Stone, J. (2020a), *Digital Play Therapy*, 1st ed., pp. 238–243.

Aiden presented for therapy with his adoptive parents. Each, including Aiden, were concerned about his outbursts of anger. Aiden expressed concerns about his anger toward his younger adoptive sibling. Further exploration revealed that Aiden was worried he would be removed from his adoptive family if his behavior did not improve, particularly toward his little brother.

Aiden's biological mother was not a reliable resource in his life and her parental rights had been terminated. His biological father died approximately a year prior to beginning treatment due to an illness.

Initial meetings with Aiden revealed that he was an intelligent, sensitive, pensive child who felt he had evil lurking within him. He stated that the evil inside came out when he was angry and he directed it toward his younger adoptive sibling. It is hypothesized that the younger sibling bore the brunt of his outbursts due to his position as the youngest in the family and presumably the one with the least amount of power amongst the siblings.

Aiden wanted to play Roblox with the therapist and overtime requested a number of different games to play. Typically the games allowed players to achieve a very high level to be perceived as superior to other players. At times Aiden would be very generous and give lower-leveled players special items which helped them level-up more quickly. Other times he reveled in destroying people's characters and/or items. It appeared to be connected to his sense of security at the time.

Within Roblox you can customize your character in numerous ways. Many players have a collection of skins and accessories which distinguish them from most other players. These components of an avatar serve as outward expressions of personality, mood, status, and more. Aiden had an extensive collection and therefore could reflect a wide variety of versions of himself.

Some readers might not be aware of the gaming platform, Roblox, so a brief description will be given here.

Roblox

Roblox is a largely misunderstood gaming platform. Adults and children alike play Roblox games. According to the Roblox website (2022), since 2018, 95.1 billion (yes, that is billion with a b) hours of the millions of available games have been played (Roblox, 2022). Roblox is internationally available and is cross platform (can be accessed from multiple devices). It includes a library of user-generated games and was founded in 2004. The premise is similar to YouTube except they provide a variety of games. In mid 2022, there were 11.1 million experiences available (Roblox, 2022). Each of the games have been created by users. The games are rated by players for game play and popularity; the more "thumbs up" a game has, the higher the rating.

The Roblox website boasts that 29.1 million developers have contributed to the game library and have been paid $1 billion (another b) for their creations (Roblox, 2022). As with other industries, the more popular a game, the higher it climbs in the ranks, and the more money the developers can make. What is unique is that developers can be of any ages and ability. Developers can create games through the Roblox Create program and the Reality Engine. In addition to professional developers and laymen developers, clients can create games with their therapist, friends, and/or their caregiver(s), or on their own.

Safety is a common and important concern regarding the use of Roblox. This is a subsection of concerns regarding online platforms and games in general. Any tool that is utilized in a therapeutic setting should be vetted for appropriate content and process. As discussed in chapter 1, therapists and the therapeutic process maintains the goal to "do no harm"; clinicians want information which allows a tool to be evaluated for use.

An investigation of the Roblox website reveals a plethora of information and resources for parents and educators. Parental controls can be activated in a number of ways, such as enacting a personal identification number (pin) or the requirement of a code which is sent to the parent's email address prior to gaining access to play. Chats are monitored with particular protections in place, such as human and autodetections, or can be completely disabled. A Roblox International Trust & Safety Advisory Board is tasked with all feature and platform issues regarding community safety (Roblox, 2022).

In therapy, the clinician will need to attend to any components regarding safety and confidentiality. A key feature when using such a tool in therapy is to have any communication, either typed or spoken, remain within the HIPAA compliant telemental health platform (i.e. Zoom) or directly to each other if in the same physical space. Additionally, profiles are best created with the client and caregivers together (as appropriate per age/ability level of client). Families would benefit from discussing concepts such as digital citizenship: how one conducts oneself online, etc. The parent section of the Roblox site provides information which could then be discussed as a family and/or within a therapeutic session.

Another therapeutic consideration has to do with public and private servers. Private servers (rooms for the creator and their invitees only) should be used when possible and appropriate. Most private servers are free of charge. While private servers provide a level of security from outside players, some game interaction relies on a particular number of players. In some situations, the therapist may want to observe, discuss, and/or intervene in multiplayer social scenarios, so playing in the public forum could be more appropriate. Understanding any risks and/or benefits of any of these games is imperative along with explaining such concerns with a minor client's caregivers.

Finally, although Roblox is a free platform, there are two types of currencies. There is an in-game currency (earned for playing, completing tasks, etc.) and real-world currency (translates to real-world cash – dollars, pounds, etc.). The in-game currency can be spent on different items depending on the game. As an example, in the game Welcome to Bloxburg, the player will be required to pay household bills. Items such as rent and utilities are paid with in-game currency and do not translate into real-world currency. Robux, the real-world currency, has a gray hexagon symbol next to it so you can be more aware of which currency is being used. Robux is another area where parental controls are important.

Self

It became apparent that Aiden's avatar in any given game was a reflection of how he was feeling that session or even moment to moment. There were times when he would maintain the same skin/appearance throughout the game play, and others where he would change skins rapidly throughout a game. There were also times when he would play the same game for the whole session each week, and others where he would want to change games before any goals were even reached.

The outward appearance of his avatar's character reflected how he was feeling about himself, his life, his relationships, and his place within this world view. Just as a client coming into session dressed in ways that contrast their typical style, i.e., a teen who typically wears bright colors and coordinated outfits begins to present in ill-fitting, mis-matched, dark clothing, might indicate a change in their functioning, avatars can indicate the same. Paying attention to the avatar, asking questions about how they feel about their avatar, what skins they wish they had, what style(s) they hope to achieve, all contributes to a deeper understanding of the client.

Of great interest is when a client is struggling with any component of their identity. How their avatar either represents the desired depiction, or represents what they feel is an expectation, greatly impacts how they feel about themselves and possibly how they present in their day-to-day life. An avatar is a bit of a projection of the person who created it, particularly in clients such as Aiden who was very invested in his avatar's appearance in each moment.

Once the therapist began to understand the meanings of his different depictions, along with coordinating the information with what was known about weekly experiences, and how he was feeling in his day-to-day life, the avatars became a bit of a litmus test and predictor of how the session might progress. The stability or rapid changing of skins and/or games was also a strong predictor. Over time the therapist queried and modeled pairing the observations with happenings in Aiden's life. Over time these observations were shared with Aiden and he began to identify the avatar's state of being, what was being reflected in the avatar's appearance, and what was going on in his day-to-day life that could be part of the avatar's representation.

References

Cooper, D. (2017, January). *The LEgend of Zelda: Breath of the Wild – Everything we know so far.* https://gamerant.com/legend-zelda-breath-of-the-wild-wiki/

Fandom (n.d., a). *History of the Legend of Zelda series.* https://zelda.fandom.com/wiki/History_of_the_Legend_of_Zelda_series

Fandom (n.d., b). *Link.* https://zelda.fandom.com/wiki/Link

Homeyer, L. & Sweeney, D. (2016). *Sandtray therapy: A practical manual.* Routledge.

Homeyer, L. & Lyles, M. (2022). *Advanced sandtray therapy: Digging deeper into clinical practice.* Routledge.

Ioannou, A., Papastavrou, E. Avraamides, M.N., & Charalambous, A. (2020). Virtual reality and symptoms management of anxiety, depression, fatigue, and pain: A systematic review. *SAGE Open Nursing, 6*, 1–13, doi: 10.1177/2377960820936163

Lowenfeld Trust (2017). *About Lowenfeld.* https://lowenfeld.org/about-lowenfeld/

Lowenfeld, M. (2007). *Understanding children's sandplay: Lowenfeld world technique.* Sussex Academic Press.

Lowenfeld, M. (1954). *Description of The Lowenfeld World Technique.* https://lowenfeld.org/wp-content/uploads/2020/09/K5-Description-of-The-Lowenfeld-World-Technique.pdf

McMahon, E. & Boeldt, D. (2022). *Virtual reality therapy for anxiety: A guide for therapists.* Routledge.

Nintendo (2017). *The Legend of Zelda Breath of the Wild: Nintendo Switch.* https://www.nintendo.com/games/detail/the-legend-of-zelda-breath-of-the-wild-switch/#game-info

Roblox (2022). *About us.* https://corp.roblox.com/

Stone, J. (2020a). *Digital play therapy: A clinician's guide to comfort and competence*, 1st ed. Routledge.

Stone, J. (2020b). The integration of play within video games in clinical practice. In A. Bean, E. Daniel, & S.A. Hayes (Eds.), *Integrating geek culture into therapeutic practice: The clinician's guide to geek therapy*. Leyline.

Stone, J. (2021a). Trauma-informed virtual reality play therapy. *Playground*, Fall/Winter, pp. 13–16.

Stone, J. (2021b). Virtual reality and play therapy with adults. *Play Therapy, 16*(4), 20–24.

9 Fear Less

Utilizing digital tools in mental health treatment is not just about using
something cool.

It's not about the newest, shiniest, and most sensational;
It's not about abandoning the fundamentals, the past, or the
concerns;

It's about understanding as much as we can
about mental health,
about humans,
about emotions,
about representation,
about honor,
about culture,
about interests,
about behavior,
about connection,
about the body,
about the brain,
about the mind,
about identity,
about ourselves,
about each other,
about our purpose,
about truth;
seeing, hearing,
accepting, understanding,
and life;

and then about
what is possible and

DOI: 10.4324/9781003171799-9

what is needed;
what we have implemented,
and what still needs to be;
it is also about
the impact
all of this can make,
and all of us can make,
for our clients,
our profession,
ourselves,
and for society.

It is about all of us
and our desire to do the very best we can
for the people who honor us
with the work
of doing all we can
to assist them
during their journey through life.

"Nothing in life is to be feared, it is only to be understood.

Now is the time to understand more, so that we may fear less".
Dr. Marie Curie

Index

autonomic nervous system (ANS) 24, 56

Central Executive Network (CEN) 67–8
Central Nervous System (CNS) 24, 31, 36, 55, 57, 61, 87
cognition 26–7, 32–3, 38, 49, 57, 60–2, 81, 86, 88, 91, 93–4
community 9, 40–3, 81, 89, 99, 105, 138
Computer-Mediated Psychotherapy (CMP) 74
concepts: abstract 20–1, 32–3, 86, 91; fundamental 11, 20
COVID-19 2, 4, 38, 98

Default Mode Network (DMN) 26, 32, 66–8, 131
digital native 73, 78
Do No Harm 6, 10–3, 18, 49, 54, 75, 79, 138

eHealth 74
embodiment 36–7, 91, 105
entertainment 8–9, 14, 74, 114
essence 6–7, 40
ethics 33, 79, 83, 86
existence 1, 16, 27, 34, 38, 42–3, 89, 91, 94, 130
Experience 3, 10, 13, 26–8, 30, 35–43, 53–4, 66, 74–7, 86, 89–92, 95–7, 101–17, 121–3, 127–35

Digital Play Therapy (DPT) 74–7, 86–95
digital tools 4–5, 7, 9, 14, 20, 49–50, 68, 71, 74, 76–9, 86, 94–7, 105, 107–8, 111, 113–116

Hippocratic Oath 10–4, 75

Identification 9, 20–3, 38, 43–4, 53–4, 76, 86–7, 89, 92, 94–5, 105, 119, 138; In-group identification 29, 4, 89
immersion 39–40, 89–90, 105, 110, 131
intention 10, 13, 27, 33–4, 50, 56, 75–6, 90, 93, 97
interoception 21–5, 33, 37, 53, 62, 66, 87, 90, 105
introspection 2, 25, 33

Metacognition 32–3, 49, 93–4
mHealth 74, 80

Neuroplasticity 30–2, 90
Neuro-rights 81–3

Perception 22, 26–8, 32–6, 40, 59, 64, 66, 86–8, 90–5, 105; depth 59; endosomatic 25; self 21–2, 28–9, 37, 87; visuospatial 60; sensory 60; speech 60
person-centered therapy 8
presence 34–6, 91; tele- 34–6, 91, 105

pretence/pretense 38–9, 92, 105
proprioception 36–7, 57, 60, 62, 91
Psychology Interjurisdictional
    Compact (PSYPACT) 4

quarantine 39, 92

reality 15, 33–5, 38–42, 52–3, 65, 67,
    89–92, 94; augmented 96, 106; Engine
    138; mixed 14, 106; virtual 14, 40, 74,
    97, 104–5, 119–121, 123, 129–132
representation 20–2, 24, 26, 29, 38–9,
    43–4, 53–4, 76, 86, 89–90, 94–5,
    105, 119, 135, 140

selective mutism 119, 123
self 87–92, 94–5, 120, 139;
    -acceptance 94; -actualization 94;
-awareness 87, 95, 105, 127–8;
-concepts 88, 91, 123; -contained
106; -identity 89, 119, 136;
-moderated 126; -other 88–9, 91,
94; -perception *see perception*;
-preservation 89, 125;
-reinforcing 121
sexual trauma 119–120
somatic nervous system (SNS) 56
standards 79, 86

Technopanic 96
Telepresence *see presence*
Theory of Mind 27, 38–9, 41, 54, 60,
    62, 66–7, 84, 88, 92, 95
Therapeutic Virtual Reality (tVR) 74

VRx 74